The Final Countdown Diet

AN INSIDER'S GUIDE TO WHY DIETS FAIL & THE SECRETS OF PERMANENT FAT LOSS

WILL MEADOWS

Published by FCD Publishing

www.finalcountdowndiet.com

First Published 2014

Copyright © Will Meadows 2014

ISBN 978-1503256071
ISBN 1503256073

To my lovely wife Jane,
for supporting me throughout.

To my wonderful children W, B & C,
for lighting up my life and teaching me more
about myself than I ever thought possible.

To Jack, the Dad taken from me before I got
to know you,
for guiding my life from the stars.

I love you all.

WILL MEADOWS

CONTENTS

DISCLAIMERS

PUBLISHER'S DISCLAIMER

The material in this book is intended solely for informational purposes only. Every person is unique and following a diet plan may not be the best course of action for you. In addition you may have health problems, diagnosed or otherwise, that could be exacerbated by following a diet plan. If in doubt you should always consult a doctor. The author and publisher expressly disclaim any responsibility for any adverse effects that may result from the use or misuse of the information and advice contained within this book.

WILL'S DISCLAIMER

You're beautiful and I don't want you to come to any harm. Consult a doctor before you diet.

WILL MEADOWS

PROLOGUE

The flight from Beijing to Bangkok had only taken about four hours. I'd been working in China for two years and was making the trip to Thailand to visit my Uncle. Mike had always been my favourite Uncle but it had been 4 years since we'd last met. Mike had moved out to Thailand shortly after my wedding to work in the construction industry and I hadn't seen him since. As we were both located in Asia I thought it would be a great opportunity to catch up with him. I had somehow overlooked the fact that we were over 2000 miles apart. For some reason Thailand just seemed to be 'next door'.

I walked out of the arrivals hall and Mike's unmistakable smile greeted me. However instead of the man-hug or handshake I was expecting, he feigned a punch to my midriff "You've got fat!" he laughed. I instinctively sucked in my stomach. "You're sucking it in now" he roared. In that moment two thoughts crossed my mind. Firstly, I wondered why on earth he was my favourite Uncle. Secondly, I realised that I had indeed 'got fat'.

In hindsight I shouldn't have been so surprised about my size. Two years of banquet-style dining in China had certainly taken their toll on my body. Unfortunately I hadn't noticed getting fat at all. My weight had literally crept up on me. I guess there were various reasons for my complete lack of awareness. However it's always good to blame misfortune on someone or something else - so I chose to blame being fat on the weather!

The seasons in China are a lot more extreme than those in Britain. The summer is hot and humid and the winter is blisteringly cold. As a result I was constantly changing clothes to cope with the seasons. Over a two-year period my clothes had got bigger as I had grown bigger. I had noticed my L frame was now an XL but I just blamed it on dodgy sizing.

The truth was the sizing was fine; my weight had slipped without me even noticing. Not only that, I could now be accurately described as 'fat' by those close to me. This is exactly how it happens for many people. You don't get overweight overnight. It's a gradual, almost imperceptible, process. It creeps up on you. Over time your clothes might not fit as well as they used to. You buy better-fitting clothes and might moan about how the shops keep altering their sizing. You may well seek out shops that have the 'right' size. The fact is the sizes and the shops haven't changed: you have.

On that day in Bangkok I made a conscious decision to get my old body back. I came to realise that I hadn't gained weight overnight and I wasn't going to lose it overnight either. I tried lots of diets and generally ended up heavier than when I began. Some diets were better than others but the fat would always pile back on. I would later discover that this wasn't my fault: it was a natural reaction of my body. I also discovered that it doesn't matter whether you are male or female – everyone's body acts in exactly the same way.

Having struggled to lose weight during my time in China, I had a stroke of luck. I was fortunate enough to receive a job offer from a UK company working with some of the biggest names in the diet industry. It was a dream job and it might just help me find a solution to my weight issues. Full of excitement I returned to the UK.

The company worked at the forefront of the diet industry. My role was to get the product onto the supermarket shelves and ensure it was effectively marketed. I won lots of awards and also discovered the tricks the diet industry uses to change the consumer's behaviour. Over time I could spot which new diets would work and which ones wouldn't.

A few years later and another job opportunity arose, this time within the sports nutrition industry. At that time sports nutrition was experiencing an immense period of growth. I had the great privilege to work in a company that was at the cutting edge of the industry. The products we produced went on to help some of the best athletes in the world.

My experience in the diet and nutrition industries helped me to develop my own diet system – the system in this book. This diet has helped myself and others to lose fat - permanently. In writing this book I wanted to tell the millions of Yo-Yo dieters around the world that it's not their fault their last diet failed. I believe that some diets are destined to fail and this book explains why.

The ultimate aim of this book however is to give you the information you need to lose fat effectively and to keep that fat off - permanently. I want this book to be the last diet book you will ever need to buy. I hope you enjoy the book.

THE BIG FAT QUESTIONS

Before we start the book proper let's begin with some easy questions. Answer the below as honestly as you can:

1. Do you want to achieve a slimmer body?
2. Do you want to lose fat?
3. Do you want to keep that fat off permanently?
4. Do you want a bikini body in 4 weeks?
5. Do you want rapid weight loss with real results in 7 days?
6. Do you want a diet that all the celebrities are mad about?

If you've answered 'Yes' to the majority of the above then you are not alone. Maybe there's a 'No' or two dotted in amongst your answers but my guess is you've picked up this book purely because the majority of the questions resonate with you. You want a better body and you want it now!

Now I'd like you to go back and think for a moment about what success in each of the above questions looks like. What would the outcome be? As an example, the successful outcome from Question One would be that you have a slimmer body.

Next I'd like you to rank those outcomes in order of importance. For example, is losing fat permanently more or less important than celebrity endorsement? Grab yourself a pen and list the outcomes that are the most important to you. Do it now – don't just skip this exercise like you were going to!

Once you've completed the above it's time for me to be brutally honest. If you think the outcomes contained in questions 1 to 3 are the most important then we can work together to make you the person you want to be. If your focus is solely on those outcomes listed in questions 4 to 6 then I'm afraid you might have picked up the wrong book - but don't put it down just yet! Hear me out.

The majority of popular diets focus on similar areas to those contained in questions 4 to 6. The problem is that the majority of those diets don't work. Let me qualify that statement. I don't think they work in the *long-term*. A lot of diets only offer short-term fixes. Sure, you might achieve rapid weight loss from, for example, drinking lemon juice for a few weeks but as soon as you start eating normal foods again the weight just piles back on.

The fact is most people tend to have a short-term focus. We want weight loss and we want it now. We therefore pick a diet that promises rapid results. If that diet tells us to drink only lemon juice or eat cabbage soup then we'll gladly do this to achieve our aim – quickly. However once the diet ends, the sad fact is that most people will put all their weight back on. If we could see ourselves in a few months time having made no progress would we make the same choices? Would we go through the 'pain' without any gain? Of course we wouldn't.

This is where our short-term focus is out of line with what we really want to achieve. In the short-term we want rapid weight loss. In the long-term we want to keep that weight off. The problem is that most diets concentrate on the short-term because it's what sells books. They promise results in '7 days' or whatever timeframe will get them noticed. Most people start these diets because they want to lose weight quickly and they want to keep that weight off. However that's not what's on offer. Many of these diets will never result in permanent weight loss[1]. There are reasons for this and these reasons are explained within the pages of this book.

Taking on board what I've just said, I'd like you to revisit the outcomes you prioritised earlier. Which are the most important to you now? Are you willing to invest a bit more time to lose fat permanently or do you still need a quick fix even though the results might not last? If you want the quick fix then I can't help you - yet. You may have perfectly good reasons for this and who am I to judge? What I will say is that the book you are holding in your hands will be there for you when you're ready to make that permanent change.

If however you have just highly ranked getting slimmer, losing fat and keeping that fat off permanently - then welcome aboard and keep reading. Your fat loss journey begins right now!

PART ONE: WHAT YOU NEED TO KNOW ABOUT LOSING FAT

The chances are that if you've bought this book you have been on a diet before. You may also have other diet books on your bookshelf. Maybe you've also bought diet foods in the past from famous brands. My guess is that all of your previous diets worked to some extent. Let me be more specific – those diets worked until something happened that led to you putting all the weight back on. I would also guess that your last diet started in January or February or sometime near the middle of the year – most likely in June or early July. Did I guess any of the above correctly?

I'm not a mind reader and these guesses aren't just simple guesses. They're educated guesses informed by my experience within the diet industry. I believe there are reasons why a large proportion of diets fail and there are reasons why you start diets at certain times of year. My search to find a better way for myself - a better diet – ultimately led to the book you're holding in your hands right now.

In this book you will hear two main terms. The first term is The Final Countdown Diet Plan ("FCD Plan"). This term covers everything contained within these pages. It consists of the information, the skills and the knowledge you need to succeed in your fat loss goals. Although the FCD Plan includes food, its principal aim is to give you an understanding of how and why successful diets work. With this information you will be better prepared to make this diet the last diet you ever need to do.

The second term introduced is the 3F System. The 3F System is all about food. The 3F System relates solely to the dietary guidance contained in the book and works in conjunction with the understanding you have gained from The FCD Plan. It is the 3F System that will help you make the mealtime choices you need to lose your body fat.

Part One of the book focuses on some of the things you should know about the world of dieting. This section opens up some of the truths about the diet industry and why a lot of diets fail. We discuss why I don't think counting calories is the best way to lose fat and why I think our bodies are naturally designed to keep hold of as much fat as they can. You need to know these things to make a success of your diet. I've not included any 'filler' in this book. Every word on every page has been written to help you achieve your fat loss aims. OK, I have attempted a few jokes along the way and you can ignore those (if you can spot them). Let's get started!

THE DIET INDUSTRY KNOWS YOU BETTER THAN YOUR MUM

Obviously for those pedants amongst you, the title of this chapter should be 'The Diet Industry Knows You Better Than Your Mum Knows You'. Instead it looks like the Diet Industry knows you quite well but isn't as well acquainted with your Mum. When I realised it could be ambiguous I thought I'd leave it in for fun. That's how much fun I am.

What do I know anyway?

How do I know what the diet industry knows about you (or your mum for that matter)? Let me tell you about some of my experience. In a career spanning two decades I held key roles in companies working in the diet and nutrition industries. I was involved in the Operational side of the businesses and was keenly involved in developing, producing and marketing products for some of the greatest diet and nutrition brands in the world.

The products I worked with made a difference to people's lives. They helped people work towards their fat loss goals and helped fuel Olympic and international success for some of the world's top athletes. In all that time I never worked with a product I didn't believe in. Everything we made and sold did exactly what we said it would. But now it's time to be honest. Some of the products I worked with would not have made much difference to you.

Just in case you were wondering – you are definitely normal

The reason why your results might be different from someone else's is simply because you are normal. Statistically of course you are more likely to be normal than a top class athlete. Similarly you are more likely to diet like a normal person compared with an actress being paid by a movie studio to lose fat for a role. My guess is you get up in the morning and go to work, or you look after the kids, do housework or do something else like studying. The chances are you don't get up and devote the rest of the day to achieving physical perfection. Athletes and actresses have the time and resources to do this however it's outside the experience of us 'normals'. Most of us have to make do with the circumstances that life brings us. As a result we are unlikely to be asked to model underwear any time soon. That doesn't make us bad people. We just have other priorities like real jobs and real families that often take precedence over looking after ourselves.

The thing is, the diet industry knows you have other priorities. They know you're busy, they know your life is hectic and they know at what times of the year you'll start thinking about looking after yourself. When those times come they 'reach out' to you through advertising. They know you'll probably be feeling a bit self-conscious and are probably looking to improve your weight. In short, they know when you'll be at your most vulnerable and they target you then. That may sound harsh but it's an industry and nobody is going to advertise all year round when they know exactly the time of year to press your buttons for maximum effect. Not only that, no matter whether you're trying to lose fat by dieting or exercise, the diet and fitness industries use exactly the same methods.

All health industries use the same tactics

After my initial job in the diet industry, I went on to take up a senior role in one of the UK's most respected Sports Nutrition companies. Part of my job was to be responsible for the Company's marketing. I was completely new to the Sports Nutrition industry. I knew that the diet industry repeated certain advertising themes throughout the year but had no idea what the sports and fitness industries did. To get up to speed quickly I decided to start by analysing the publications we'd be advertising in. I took 5 year's worth of magazines off the shelf, from a variety of health and fitness titles, and laid them all out on the floor arranging them by month of issue (granted, this was a bit OCD). I then wrote down the main cover stories from each magazine for each month and input them into a spreadsheet so I could sort and arrange them by subject (definitely OCD!). So what did all this activity tell me?

What I discovered was that over a 5-year period the same topics were repeated over and over again – at exactly the same time of year. Not only that, competing magazines would run stories covering identical subjects – in exactly the same month. With this information I was able to create an advertising calendar to identify which products we should be advertising at which times of year. This would tie in with the overall theme of the magazines. People would buy the magazines because they had a specific aim and then find an advert for one of our products that would help them to achieve that aim. The plan worked and it put us ahead of the competition. Sales at the Company increased by 20% year after year. The fact is that advertising works when it offers something to the consumer that fulfils a need. We had what we believed were the best products on the market and it made sense to make people aware of our products when they were looking to achieve certain aims.

Diet when it's good for you, not when it's good for 'them'

Why am I telling you this? Because I think it's important that when you start a diet you do it at a time that's good for you and when your mind is set on achieving your aims. You should never start a diet because some magazine or advertisement tells you to. In addition, the messages sent out at certain times of year by some diet companies are simply unachievable: 'Rapid results!' 'Fast weight loss!' 'A Bikini Body in 4 weeks!'. What happens when you reach the 4-week point and don't achieve that aim? Are you a failure? Absolutely not! You have been set up to fail and it's not your fault. The diet you were following was never going to work and its goals were impossible. You therefore should only start a diet when the time's right for you and you need to ignore the hype at the key dieting periods. What's more, you don't need to invest in any special dietary food to achieve diet success.

The guidelines within this book will help you to achieve consistent achievable fat loss without resorting to any special 'quick fix' diet food. Let's face it; there is something wrong when you can buy diet food in the supermarket on a Buy-One-Get-One-Free basis. They're positively encouraging you to eat more! The key is to stick with the programme in this book and keep at it no matter what external pressures you might face. At specific times of the year the claims of the latest fad diet may seduce you. My belief is that if you resort to one of these diets you will end up back at square one. The reasons why I believe this can be found in the *How Your Brain Keeps You Fat* chapter later in this book. So how do you know when you are being 'seduced' by the big diet companies?

Use your own calendar, not theirs

The messages sent out by the big diet companies can be very persuasive. The offers seem too good to miss. But you mustn't jump on the bandwagon and go for the quick fix diet that's sure to fail. You must only diet when the time is right for you and you need to remain focussed on the main goal of long-term and sustainable fat loss. So you can prepare yourself for those times when the external pressure to lose weight is at its most intense, here is what the diet industry calendar looks like:

January – The biggest month of the year. Everyone has eaten to excess over Christmas and the New Year's Resolutions are clocking up. In January you can't move for diet plans on TV, healthy eating offers in supermarkets and gym 'taster sessions' being thrown at you. It's boom time for the diet industry and chances are this is when you've done most of your dieting in the past.

March/April – typically around Easter there's another, smaller, burst of activity. Some people will be going away on holiday and want to look their best. Maybe they're trying on their swimsuits and have noticed they're a bit more snug than usual. Maybe they've over indulged on Easter eggs! No matter the reason the diet industry is there to 'help'. New products appear on supermarket shelves and advertising picks up again after the post January lull.

July/August – now we're really into the holiday season.

Magazines scream at you to get a 'Bikini Body'. Typically you're also told that the body of your dreams can be achieved in only 4 to 6 weeks. Pictures of overweight celebrities in bikinis grace the cover of some magazines and you might also get some B-list 'star' telling you how they achieved their remarkable new slender figure (which is probably linked to some product they're trying to sell and won't mention the personal trainer they've had camped out in their house for the last 6 months)

September gives you another chance to get that Beach Ready Body in a last ditch attempt to sweep up those punters who don't have kids so can holiday outside of school time. It's also a time when the diet companies prick the conscience of those people who failed to reach this goal in the July/August period.

From October to November the diet industry is pretty quiet. They know that Christmas is coming up and now it's just a waiting game. They're happy to sit by and let you over-indulge knowing that you'll be guilty as Hell in January and the calendar can start all over again.

Believe it or not, these themes are repeated each year without fail. You have to wonder why you get a second chance at that Beach Body. Is it because they knew you were never going to get it in the first place?

This constant churning of diet advice and the pressure to jump on-board the latest 'fad' diet creates a vicious cycle: the Yo-Yo Diet we all know about. This is ultimately why I wrote this book, to get you out of the Yo-Yo Dieting cycle. I also wanted to provide a real alternative to losing fat that didn't rely on unnecessary traditional dieting methods. The first such method we will consider is the apparent need to count every single calorie you consume.

WHY COUNTING CALORIES DOESN'T WORK

First a definition: **"Calorie** (kal-oh-ree) *n.* a tiny pixie that lives in your wardrobe and sews your clothes tighter every night".

OK, that might not be a precise definition but it just about sums up what most of us think about calories. Calories rule our world and are to blame for all sorts of things that make us feel bad about ourselves - this includes making our clothes feel tighter. Calories are the guys who tell you to calm down when you're having fun. They tell you what to eat and they make you feel guilty when you don't listen. Here's the thing, you don't need to count calories to get slimmer.

Many diets start with an assumption that you are quite happy recording the calorie intake of every meal you consume. The problem is this soon gets *very, very* boring. To get around our very low boredom thresholds, some companies give you an app which basically automates things until the novelty wears off. What these diets and app-makers are missing is that calories are only part of the story. Not only that, there's an assumption that all calories are equal and it's just a matter of eating fewer to get slimmer. However here's the big secret: not all calories were created equal.

Not all calories are the same

Let's assume the following. I have in front of me a nice big plate of chicken curry with a bit of rice and veg on the side. I take out my smartphone and input all the details about this meal into my calorie counting app. There are 800 calories on my plate. As a main meal that's not too bad. Now let's assume that instead of my nice curry I have simply poured the equivalent calorific amount of sugar onto my plate (incidentally this is about 200g of sugar). Do you think this will affect my body in the same way? The science backing up calorie-driven diets tells me that it must do. 800 calories are 800 calories regardless. In fact, a calorie-driven diet tells me that if I eat another 2 plates of sugar I will be just below my daily calorific intake target and will lose fat. The sugar diet! What could be better? Of course this would be nonsense.

So why are 800 calories of sugar different from 800 calories of curry? The answer is that when I eat sugar all it gives me is energy. Nothing else. Sugar does not contain any nutrients, vitamins or minerals. After the meal my body will detect I've just pigged out on a plate of sugar and will release a hormone called insulin whose job is to try to find somewhere to stick all this sugar. Insulin does this because it knows that sugar is toxic and my body can't possibly use all of that sugar as energy. Unfortunately insulin only knows two places to store the sugar. One place it can put it is in our Glycogen fuel tank where it will store it to be used as energy later on. However the problem is that the Glycogen fuel tank can only hold so much. This means that the insulin has to opt for Plan B – which is to store the sugar in another place. That other place is our fat cells. That's where all the excess sugar is going: straight to fat.

Sugar is both simple and complex!

My curry meal on the other hand presents my body with a range of nutrients that are essential to keep me healthy and alive. My plate also contains some sugar. However the sugars in the curry act a bit differently. Whereas standard sugar is called a simple carbohydrate, the sugars within rice and vegetables are called complex carbohydrates. Unlike the plate of simple sugar I ate earlier these complex sugars contain both nutrients and energy. Critically, the energy they provide doesn't immediately enter the blood to end up in our fat cells. The energy from complex carbohydrates gets released more slowly. It drips into our bloodstream helping to maintain a nice and even level of energy.

The slow release of energy from complex carb is the complete opposite of the energy spike we get from simple sugars. During my time working for the sports nutrition company we used simple sugars in products designed specifically to give top international cyclists an energy boost. Such sugars are ideal when you're on a 100-mile race and are just approaching the bottom of a punishing mountain. In such circumstances you need simple sugars and the extra energy they provide. The sad fact is that most of us will never expend that much energy. For us, those simple sugars will inevitably become fat.

Sugar is great at hide and seek

'Why are you telling me all this?' I hear you complain 'I'm not stupid enough to eat a plate of sugar'. I know you're not - the problem is that sugar hides in many forms. You may well end up eating the equivalent of a plate of sugar and not realise it. Some sugars are easy to spot. The sugar in an energy drink or in a can of Cola is pretty obvious to spot. Other sugars tend to hide themselves a bit better and are less well publicised. If something is called 'syrup' it's basically a runny sugar. If something ends in 'ose' it's also a sugar (look for fructose, glucose, lactose, maltose etc.). Even seemingly natural ingredients are loaded with sugar. Look out for sugars described as corn sweetener, honey, molasses etc. They might sound innocent: but they're deadly.

One simple way to reduce the amount of bad sugars you are ingesting is to have a look at a food label. Try to do this before you eat the contents of the packet! Better still, do this before you buy the product in the first place. The food laws in most countries require manufacturers to list food ingredients in the proportion they appear in the finished product. The higher up an ingredient is on the list - the more of it there is in the product. Obviously if the ingredient declaration lists 'sugar' as the second ingredient a) it's dead easy to spot and; b) a high proportion of your meal is going to go straight to fat. Take note of the ingredient lists on the foods you buy and try to avoid anything with a sugar in the top 3 main ingredients. Processed foods such as ready meals tend to be loaded with sugars. Avoid processed foods whenever you can.

Look for sugar instead of calories

Why so much talk about sugar? Firstly, we need to have an awareness of where our calories come from rather than just blindly noting how many calories we consume. Secondly, it's likely that we actually have more control over restricting sugars than we have over restricting calories. When we grab some food on the go or dine out the calorific information is not always readily available. How many calories does that plate of Chicken Chow Mein have? Who knows? We can however generally make an educated guess at which choice on the menu will be loaded with sugar – think Sweet & Sour Chicken versus Stir Fried Chicken. The Stir Fried option is likely to contain less sugar than chicken with a sweetened sauce. One way therefore to avoid the food you eat going straight to fat is to restrict your sugar intake rather than simply count the calories.

Another problem arises when you rely solely on counting calories. Cutting calories often results in your body being denied essential vitamins, minerals and energy. When your body senses it is being denied nutrients it responds by holding on to the fat it already has. When this happens your brain also gets in on the act and makes sure you start to find food even more appealing than normal. This brain activity will be covered later in the book but for now we need to consider the main classes of nutrients that are essential for a healthy and balanced diet.

Getting the nutritional balance right

You need to know about nutrients. I had no idea what they were until I was way into my mid-30s. By then it was too late and I was piling the fat on. The reason I didn't want to know anything about nutrients was because I thought they were boring. I now realise they are far from boring and an understanding of the main nutrients will make all the difference to whether or not you'll lose fat. The groups you need to know about are proteins, carbohydrates, fats, fibre, vitamins, minerals and water. You cannot get all of these from one single food source so a balanced diet is essential.

Proteins: they'll fix you up good

First up are proteins. Think of proteins like a little first aid kit solely for your body. The body needs protein to repair and maintain itself and to perform basic bodily functions. Your hair, nails, skin, muscles and bones all contain protein. Proteins are also particularly important at key stages of growth and development such as childhood, puberty and pregnancy. Simply put, they help your body to fix itself (this will fall into place later on). However, not all proteins are created equal and some are absorbed and put to use by the body more readily. Good sources of protein are egg whites, milk, beef, soya beans, tuna, chicken, lentils, peanuts and rolled oats[2]. We do however need to be careful when choosing our protein-packed foods. Some protein-rich foodstuffs, such as milk and rolled oats, also contain high levels of carbohydrates which we need to keep an eye on.

Carbohydrates: fuel for your tank

We have already met Carbohydrates ("carbs") in our earlier discussion when I wondered whether to eat a plate of curry or just stick with sugar. To recap, carbs principally come in two different types: Simple and Complex. All carbohydrates contain sugar. Simple carbs contain one or two units of sugar and Complex carbs contain three or more units of sugar. Even though there is more sugar in a complex carb, as we discussed earlier, a complex carb will release its sugar more slowly than a simple carb. This means you will avoid the energy spike you get from simple carbs and the sugar you consume is less likely to go straight to your fat cells. So, how do we fit carbohydrates into our balanced diet?

You will have heard a lot about low carb diets. I believe that some of these diets can be very restrictive. Instead of eating a whole range of nutrients you end up living a carnivore's fantasy where protein is the key nutrient and the only thing on the menu is meat, meat and more meat. I believe it makes more sense to consider the *type* of carbs we put into our bodies rather than just take a blanket approach and label all carbs as bad. We know that sugars are not good for us and we should therefore try to exclude highly processed foods as they typically contain lots of sugar. If we exclude such processed foods our resultant daily intake of carbs is likely to come from: flour-based products, whole grains, beans & legumes, pasta, fruit, vegetables and most soft drinks. Some of these have higher carb levels than others and we need to be careful about the quantity of the high carb foods we consume.

It's all about density

How do we know what is 'high carb'? Some scientists believe that there is a point at which a carb becomes 'bad'. One hypothesis suggests that good carbs have a carbohydrate density of below 23%[3]. Carbohydrate density is found by subtracting the amount of fibre from the total carbohydrate amount. As an example, if you look up the nutritional information for a sweet potato online you will find that there are 27g of carbohydrates and 3g of fibre per

100g of sweet potato. Now all you need to do is subtract the carbs from the fibre to give a carbohydrate density of 24g (27g − 3g = 24g). Because all the information is based on 100g of sweet potato you automatically have a percentage of 24%. This is slightly above the identified 'good carb' cut off point of 23%. The aim is to limit your intake of those foods with a carb density above 23%.

The rationale for limiting your intake of foods above 23% is that lower density carbs get released slowly into the bloodstream whereas foods with higher densities (above 23%) such as flour, sugar, grains, processed foods and certain vegetables will hit the bloodstream at higher levels than our bodies are designed to cope with. This results in weight gain − even if you are following a traditional low carb diet. This may be one explanation for why low carb dieters hit a plateau after an initial period of rapid weight loss and then slowly start to put the weight back on again. Let's now move away from carbs and consider fats.

Fats: the big fat truth

"Fat" - the very name and the very idea conjures up bad images. Walk into any supermarket and the shelves are full of low fat foods. Invariably you will find these in the healthy living section. This has to mean that fats are bad. Right? The more fats you eat the fatter you'll become. Right? As with many things - it's not that simple. Even though many of us now routinely choose the low fat version of our favourite foods this has not resulted in a slimmer society. A study in the American Journal of

Medicine[4] discovered an interesting trend. It found that over a 15-year period the fat intake of the US population had dropped by 11%. We might assume that the logical outcome would be a slimmer nation. However obesity rates over the same period had actually *increased* by 31%. How could this be so?

Fats don't make you fat

One reason that obesity has risen may well be the fact that it is actually quite difficult to remove fat from some foods whilst keeping them tasty. My time in the diet food business taught me that when you take out fat you have to put something else back in to stop the food from tasting bland. That something is usually our old enemy: sugar. The added sugar results in high levels of energy which tend to go straight to fat. Another American study found that women who followed a low fat diet didn't experience any more, or less, weight loss than those on a 'normal' diet. Put another way, eating fat doesn't make you fat[5].

In fact, your body needs fat. It provides a good source of energy and helps your body absorb lots of vitamins such as vitamins A, D, E and K that are important to your health. You might have heard about the benefits of Omega-3 and Omega-6 and how important they are for helping your body to function properly. These are known as essential fatty acids. Omega-3 can be found in certain types of fish (e.g. salmon, herring, sardines and tuna) and commercially produced fish oil tablets. Such essential fatty acids are particularly important for things like brain development (which is why the old wives tale of fish being 'Brain Food' is actually spot on), and for supporting the immune system. Omega-6 carries many of the same health benefits and can be found in things like Olive Oil, Green Vegetables and Nuts & Seeds. The thing is you have to *eat* these essential fatty acids. Your body can't make them on its own. It therefore stands to reason that you need fat in your diet.

Fibre: cleansing, filling, slimming

Now on to Fibre (or Fiber as our American friends know it). Fibre does lots of good things. You'll probably have heard that it's good for your bowels (keeps you regular etc.) but it can also help you to feel full. That's obviously great if you want to lose fat because if you feel full you'll probably want to eat less food. Fibre comes in two basic types: soluble and insoluble. The difference between the two types relates to what happens to them when they're passing through your bowel. Soluble fibre is broken down by the bacteria in your bowel and insoluble fibre is...er....insoluble. As such, it doesn't get broken down by the processes of digestion and passes through you largely the same as when it went in. Both types of fibre are good for you. Insoluble fibre is good for the health of your bowel. It's like a Scouring Pad slowly cleaning up your tubes as it passes through (now there's a nice mental image!). Soluble fibre is also good for your bowel and can additionally lower cholesterol.

Taking it slow

Importantly for our purposes, when you eat fibre it helps to slow down the absorption of carbs into your blood. We discussed earlier that if you eat too many carbs at once they inevitably end up being stored as fat. However eating the same carbs with fibre will result in the sugar being released over a longer period of time. This gives you the chance to burn it off as energy instead of it getting stored as fat. Fibre also helps you to feel fuller for longer so you won't eat as much later in the day. This satiating effect combined with the slow energy release is incredibly useful if you want to get slimmer.

There are various sources of fibre available to us. Insoluble fibres can be found in breakfast cereals, brown rice and fruit and vegetables (broccoli is a great addition to any meal as it ensures you get a significant fibre 'hit'). Soluble fibres can be found in beans, lentils and other pulses as well as in oats. Next on the 'must have' list of things to consume are vitamins and minerals.

Vitamins & Minerals: from food not a bottle

Vitamins and minerals do lots of different things to keep your body healthy. For example, they help you to see properly in dim light, they help build strong bones and teeth, they help your immune system and they protect your body from damage. No single food source contains them all so it's important that you have a balanced diet with a good variety of foods. If you feel that you may be missing out on any class of vitamins you may be tempted to take a supplement however it's not really necessary. If you follow the guidance in this book you'll be eating a healthy and balanced diet and will not be deficient in any vitamin or mineral. That's all you need to do. No pill popping, no rattling tubs to carry around with you, just follow the guidance in these pages and you'll be OK.

Water works!

Now on to the final thing in our list: Water! We all know water is good for us. It's more rehydrating than virtually anything else, it restores all the fluids we've lost through sweating and breathing and it doesn't contain any calories. It also costs nothing straight from the tap. Few of us however habitually walk around with a glass or bottle of water in our hands. This may well be because water itself is pretty boring. I try to liven up my water by adding something to it. This might be a slice of lemon or lime for example. This is often enough to make a glass of water more interesting to drink. Please however avoid going for the easy option of choosing a store-bought bottle of water that comes with a 'hint' of some fruit flavour or another. You'll find when you look on the label that these products tend to be loaded with sugars. It's far better to make your own. It also costs less and is fresher.

In this chapter we've discussed that relying solely on counting calories is pretty nonsensical. We've identified sugars as the real bad guys and spoken about how it's important to include a whole range of nutrients, including fats and carbohydrates, within a balanced diet. This information will be useful for the next chapter which considers how your brain and body reacts you start a 'traditional' diet. We will discover that your body is pretty efficient at putting fat back on. In fact it's designed that way.

IN A NUTSHELL

- Not all calories are equal. The source of the calorie is initially more important than the quantity.

- Limiting sugar is more important than limiting calories. Sugar contains no nutrients and has a high chance of ending up as fat.

- Sugar comes in many forms and is known by many names. Generally ending in 'ose'.

- Proteins are the first aid kit of our body. They help us to thrive. Good sources come from foods such as eggs, beef, chicken, tuna, lentils and oats.

- Carbohydrates come in two basis forms. Simple and Complex. Try to avoid simple carbs and opt for complex ones as they release their sugars more slowly.

- Try to limit those foods that have high carbohydrate densities.

- Fats have had a bad press but you need them in your

diet.

- Fibre is great. It helps your bowel stay healthy and reduces the rate at which carbs are absorbed into your bloodstream. It also makes you feel full so you won't need to eat as much.

- You can get vitamins and minerals from a balanced diet. You don't have to pop any pills.

- Water is vital to keep our body fluids topped up. Liven up your water with a slice of something to make it more interesting to drink.

HOW YOUR BRAIN KEEPS YOU FAT

If you've ever dieted only to find that the weight has piled back on afterwards – you are not alone. Most dieters will, over the long-term, regain the weight they have lost[6]. This reality is actually built into the business plans of some diet companies. In fact it is so commonplace they make lots of money out of it.

I once sat in a business meeting with one of the World's biggest and most successful diet companies. Their business is based around groups of people getting together to weigh themselves and receive diet advice. This company informed me that a significant proportion of their income came from members who didn't turn up anymore but were still paying subscriptions. They even had a term for them: 'inactive members'.

During our discussion, a profile of these 'inactive members' emerged. The member tended to be female. She had joined the programme, attended the meetings and had experienced some weight loss. Over time however she had put the weight back on. As a result she no longer felt comfortable being weighed in public. Maybe she felt like she had failed. However she still continued to pay her monthly subscription because 'one day' she planned to start losing weight again. This is very sad.

You are basically a caveman/woman (in better shoes)

When starting a diet, the first thing you must understand is that your body has been programmed through millions of years of evolution to hold on to fat. It's a caveman/woman thing and there's nothing you can do to stop it. If you think about the evolution of humankind it's historically been better to be fat than it is to starve to death. Food was often scarce for long periods and if you've got one fat guy and one thin guy sat in a cave without food you know which one will survive the winter! Our brains however have no idea that things have changed and don't realise that in the modern developed world you're more likely to die from obesity-related issues than you are from starvation. If we're hungry we can dial a Pizza; however our body doesn't know that food is only a phone call away. We therefore have no option but to live with the tools our bodies have developed to hold on to fat. These tools are not going to change for at least another few thousand years – if they ever change at all.

Your body knows exactly what you should weigh

All is not lost though; despite what you may think your body does quite a good job of keeping your weight stable. Some days you might delicately nibble at a selection of healthy snacks and on other days it's like feeding time at the zoo. Even though your food intake varies quite a lot, over time your body weight will more or less remain constant. Obviously if you start starving yourself or over-feeding for a lengthy period this will have a negative impact. The reason your body can keep your weight stable is because it has a baseline weight. This is the weight that your body thinks you should weigh[7]. The good news is that this baseline weight can change over time. The bad news is that the baseline tends to get heavier rather than lighter. To further rub Maldon Sea Salt into the wounds the baseline is more efficient at protecting us *against* weight loss than it is at preventing weight gain.

Survival of the fattest

If we go back to those guys sat in the cave, it would make great sense for their bodies to hold on to fat during the long winter months when food is scarce. This is their body protecting them against weight loss. It would also make sense for their bodies to take advantage of every feeding opportunity to put a bit of fat aside for the rest of the winter. This is their body helping them to gain weight. Although such mechanisms are of little help in the modern world, we have no option but to accept that this is how we have evolved as humans. It is the way humankind was built and it's the reason you and I are sat here today. If our ancestors didn't have this mechanism they would have starved to death when food supplies ran scarce. That would be the end of our family tree and there would be no you and I. So although we may not like it – at least we're around to not like it!

Eat less and you burn less

The brain uses several tricks to ensure your weight is maintained at your baseline level and to protect you from starving. One trick is to reduce your body's Basal Metabolic Rate ("BMR") when you begin eating less. The BMR is the amount of energy your body uses when you're sitting still, lying down or sleeping. It's the minimum amount of calories your body uses to keep you going without burning any calories for movement. Reducing the BMR makes sense if you're hibernating over the winter but doesn't make sense if you're living a normal daily life and simply eating less. The result of the brain's action in lowering your BMR is that even though you're consuming fewer calories, you are also *burning* fewer calories. Not only this, to encourage you to start eating more your brain tricks you into finding food more tempting than it normally is. But your brain doesn't stop there - it has other tricks up its sleeve.

Leptin the fat messenger

Your brain receives signals from a hormone within

your body called Leptin. This hormone floats around in your blood and its job is to tell your brain how much fat is in your body. Leptin is released into your blood by your fat cells. This is fine until you start losing body fat. Less fat means less Leptin is released. Your brain receives the 'Leptin levels are lower' signal and panics. It wants to restore Leptin levels and the only way it can think of doing this is to make you hungry so you'll eat more[8]. Not only that, a study in Australia[9] found evidence to suggest that your brain also pushes you towards eating high calorie food whilst simultaneously increasing the sense of 'reward' you feel after eating such food. This consumption of high calorie food combined with a lowering of your BMR will result in you putting fat on. This process continues until your Leptin levels stabilise (i.e. you've put the fat back on) and your brain tells your body that it can stop feeding.

However, the long-term overweight have to face another problem. Over the long-term, consistently high fat levels produce correspondingly high Leptin levels. This forces the brain in such people to overload to such an extent that it can't respond properly to the Leptin signals being sent. This results in what is known as 'Leptin resistance'. What happens in Leptin resistant people is that although the brain receives signals saying "Hey, fat levels are fine, no need to keep on eating" it can't understand what is being said and instead opts for the 'safe' approach and decides to make that piece of cake look *really* appetising. Evil is not the word!

Leptin's a better fighter than you

If you have a thin guy and a large guy starting out on a calorie restrictive diet both of their bodies will do everything possible to pile that lost fat back on at the first opportunity. It doesn't matter what weight these guys start out at. Trying to lose fat simply by cutting calories is forcing you to fight your body's biology. As a species we will be able to lick our elbows (try it!) before this biology changes so there is no point in trying to fight it. At this point in time there is also no magic Leptin pill that can stop your brain from making you eat when you don't need to. We therefore need to take matters into our own hands and consider ways in which we can lose fat without drastically affecting Leptin levels. Luckily, The Final Countdown Diet has been designed to do just that. Keep reading!

IN A NUTSHELL

- Your body has evolved to be an efficient fat storage machine.

- Your body is generally efficient at keeping your weight stable although this baseline weight can change over time.

- Unfortunately the baseline weight tends to increase rather than decrease.

- Your brain's job is to protect you from starving. It does this by lowering the level of energy you burn and by making all foods seem really attractive.

- The brain monitors your body's fat levels via Leptin

signals. If low fat levels are detected the brain makes you hungry and pushes you towards high calorie food.

- If you continue to be overweight your brain stops hearing the Leptin signals and tells your body to keep on eating.

EXERCISE: THE INEFFICIENT FAT
BURNER

Exercise is great for your body. "Tell me something I don't know" you say. The thing is, we all *know* exercise is good but how many of us actually *do* it? Go to any gym in January and it's packed to the rafters with people sweating away or being 'inducted' into how to use the latest torture (sorry, 'fitness') equipment. There will often be a queue for the treadmills and the whole experience is a bit noisy and smelly. Go to the same gym in April and it'll be empty. You can have your pick of the machines and the whole atmosphere is far more pleasant. So why isn't it busier in April? My guess is that many of those people who joined in January did so because they wanted to lose weight. With an empty gym 4 months later there can only be two possible outcomes: they've either achieved their weight loss aim (so don't need to exercise anymore) or they've failed and given up. My guess is it's typically the second outcome.

More exercise = more food

What those gym goers in January didn't realise is that exercise is a pretty inefficient way of trying to lose fat. Here's why. When we undertake a large amount of strenuous exercise this uses up a lot of energy. Our body senses this energy is lost and attempts to replace it. There is only one way it can do this – it makes you extremely hungry. Ever heard of the phrase 'working up an appetite'? That is exactly what you are doing when you exercise to excess. Very few of those January gym goers will have gone to the gym thinking they're just going to do a few gentle exercises and build up from there. Most of them will have completely 'kicked the backside' out of their workout sessions and will have emerged from the gym a huffing and puffing sweaty mass. Their body responds to this exertion by directing them to the nearest snack. Unfortunately, it's very difficult to resist the desire to eat in this situation. We will consider the effect of willpower later in this book however, for now, all we need to know is that it is almost impossible to fight this hunger over the long-term.

Exercise is moderately good for you

Moderate exercise is however of benefit to you in losing fat. Here's the bit where I tell you I'm not a Doctor and before you embark on any fitness plan you need to consult a medical practitioner to ensure it's right and safe for you. I'm also not an airline pilot so please don't get on a plane if I'm the only other person on-board. Anyway, what do I mean by moderate exercise? This is exercise where you're a little bit out of breath but not huffing, puffing, panting, feeling dizzy and wishing it was all over. You will be surprised to find that simple changes to your activity levels will make a difference to the amount of fat you lose. Because we're talking about small incremental changes here you won't be working up a raging hunger. Nor will you be embarking on an extreme fitness regime that you're unlikely to keep up.

Take the stairs

What kind of exercise can be called 'moderate'? Well, really it's exercise without exercising. If you're one of those people who sits in the lounge and sends the kids or your partner upstairs to get whatever you've left behind in the bedroom – then get off your backside and get it yourself! Walking up and down the stairs is excellent exercise (what do you think those step machines in the gym are based on?) and it doesn't take long at all. I live in a house spread out over 3 floors and my wife is always asking me to go up 2 flights of stairs to get something she's left behind. I could look on this as a total imposition but I don't. I view this as 'free' exercise and I often run up the stairs. It also helps that I'm too afraid to say 'no' to her.

Hit the pavement

Here's something I've never told anyone before. There's a young woman I often see walking around the roads where I live. She's a larger lady and she's clearly walking for exercise as she always carries a water bottle. Come rain or shine she's out there in the evening walking the pavement. She's literally taking those first steps to losing weight. Every time I see her I want to stop the car (because inevitably I'm the one taking the easy route) and tell her what an inspiration she is. Of course I have never stopped the car and will never say anything because I'm scared I might unintentionally offend her. However it makes me feel good to think that one-day I *might* have that conversation. I therefore spend the rest of my journey imagining the conversation we'd have and feeling quite pleased with myself. The fact is I will never stop the car; I'm the coward and she's the brave one.

Walk don't run

Anyway, the point of all this is that going for a pleasant stroll is another easy way to expend energy without the accompanying raging hunger. You may not be aware, but the difference in energy burnt between running and walking isn't all that great. A study in America[10] measured the amount of energy expended (in kilojoules) by groups of people engaged in running and walking activities. They found that running only used 26% more energy over a set distance of 1600m. Obviously walking the distance means that this energy is burnt over a longer period. This is *exactly* what you need to stop your body switching to hunger mode. In addition, walking is less stressful on the body that running and doesn't require any special gear to do it. When you feel you want to burn a bit more energy all you have to do is walk a bit further.

Here's another reason for walking, in a study conducted in the USA a group of people were given a lemon & lime drink containing the 'hidden' sugar fructose. The effects of physical activity and inactivity were then measured. It was found that those who were inactive very quickly started to show higher cholesterol levels. Some even showed the early signs of insulin resistance – the precursor to Type 2 diabetes[11]. Those who exercised however maintained their cholesterol and blood sugar at normal levels. What is remarkable about the study is that the levels of activity undertaken were minimal. This wasn't formal gym-based exercise. It was just moving around a bit more. Typically it would be in the form of parking the car a bit further away from work and walking the remaining distance - or other activities such as taking the stairs instead of the elevator.

Still need convincing? Another study[12] tracked the weight loss of 40 obese women over 16 weeks. These ladies were divided into two groups. One group was put on a diet and given aerobic exercise; the other group went on the diet and were given moderate lifestyle changes such as walking to the shops etc. Guess what happened? Over the course of the 16-week study the amount of weight lost didn't vary much at all between the groups. The aerobic group lost 3.8kg and the lifestyle group lost 4.2kg. Cholesterol levels within both groups were also about the same. There was a follow up on both groups a year later and unfortunately both groups had regained weight. However it was the lifestyle group that had regained the least weight. One possible reason for the reduced weight gain is that it's easier to continue with small changes to your lifestyle than it is to keep attending aerobic classes. So, get out there and walk!

Be a fidget

Here's another surprising way to lose fat. Fidgeting. What? Yes, fidgeting! Before you throw the book down in a fit of incredulity – hear me out. There is a scientific term for the effect of things like fidgeting and it is 'non exercise activity thermogenesis'. What this means is basically any activity that isn't exercise but results in burning energy. Researchers have found that such activity can lessen the effects of any weight gain resulting from over-eating. In a study conducted in the USA[13] a team of scientists measured the energy expended by 24 individuals of various ages and body weights. They measured the energy when they were stood or sat motionless and then measured it again when the participants were allowed to fidget (tapping hands/feet or idly swinging legs over the side of the chair etc.). They found that fidgeting resulted in *substantial* increases in energy expenditure. Now, do I want you to sit in a corner flailing your hands around and twitching away until your friends or colleagues think you're having some kind of seizure? Obviously not. However research has shown that even the smallest things can make a difference so why not tap your foot when you hear a song on the radio? Any energy expended is a good thing.

Make your exercise marginal

I bet you're thinking how on earth you're ever going to lose fat by doing all this little stuff. In some respects you might be justified for thinking that way. It does after all go against the grain – lose fat by not doing much. It doesn't make sense does it? Actually, I think it makes a lot of sense. Here's why. Let's consider another group of people who are trying to reach their goals – athletes. I realise you are probably not an athlete but hear me out. For a world class athlete the difference between beating the other guy in a race is often measured in milliseconds. What makes this difference? Is it something massive like having the longest legs on earth or the biggest wheels on your bike? No, it's the little things that make the difference. In fact, the coaching staff behind elite athletes have a term for it. They call it 'Marginal Gains'.

Believe it or not I once sat in a meeting with a coach whose job title was the 'Director of Marginal Gains'. I imagined that his job consisted solely of doing small things of little consequence. I thought this was great and wished I had his job! However my amusement soon vanished when I realised his role carried massive responsibility. What this guy did was to search out and aggregate all the small improvements that could be made to improve an athlete's performance. He looked at their nutrition, their mental health, how they trained, what equipment they used etc. With all this information he then started to make miniscule changes. These changes were probably hardly noticeable by the athlete. They just got told to do something a slightly different way. Put together however this 'sum of marginal gains' would result in that millisecond advantage over their nearest competitor. Or put another way, the difference between Gold and Silver: the difference between being a Hero or a Zero.

Think small before you think big

Now, I understand that you are not a top-level athlete. Neither am I. However small changes do make a difference. In fact, small changes are easier to make for the very reason that they are so small. Walking to the local shops instead of driving is both easy and preferable to going to the gym three times a week. Incorporating a stroll into your life is also easier and more sustainable than training for a marathon.

I hope I have shown you that the small things *do* make a difference and I would encourage you, when considering exercise, to think small before you think big. There will be time to run marathons and climb mountains or whatever you might want to do in the future but for now sustainability is the key. It's the small things that will make the biggest impact. To paraphrase what the Dalai Lama once said, "if you don't think small things matter – try sleeping in a room with a mosquito!"

IN A NUTSHELL

- Exercise is an inefficient way to lose fat because it causes your body to want more food.

- Small changes to your activity levels will help you lose fat without the hunger.

- Going for a walk or taking the stairs is enough to result in positive health benefits.

- Fidgeting can help you lose fat – but you might look a bit odd.

- The key thing to remember is that if you do lots of little things they will all add up to a big result.

PART TWO: LET'S TALK ABOUT FOOD

If you've just jumped to this page without reading all the other stuff that goes before it then shame on you! Admittedly that's *just* the sort of thing that I would do however having written the first part of the book I can positively tell you that it's full of stuff that you need to know. By all means, read this section to find out about the food choices you need to make however please, please, please go back to the start of the book and give your brain the information it really needs to make this diet a success.

In the first part of the book we covered some of the problems you are going to face when you try to lose fat. We considered the drawbacks of simply counting calories and why exercise isn't a fat loss solution in itself. We also outlined how millions of years of evolution have led to our bodies becoming supreme fat storage machines.

This second part of the book outlines an eating plan that will address some of the problems of this evolutionary hurdle. This eating plan is called the 3F System. The 3F system does not rely on counting calories but instead helps you to make sensible food choices without some of the drastic changes required by 'starvation' dieting systems. At this stage it is probably useful to highlight some of the pitfalls of other dieting systems that are avoided by following the 3F System.

Why exactly did your last diet fail?

Thus far in this book we've covered real physiological reasons why some diets will never work. These physiological factors are things that happen within your body that will prevent you from losing fat. I'm not going to go over these again but instead want to highlight some of the impracticalities of most diet systems that will set you up to fail from the outset.

The first major fail of most diet systems is that they're too rigid. It's "their way or the highway". When you engage with such a strict diet you feel like you're being denied the very things that you love eating. Most people who are denied something tend to want that 'something' even more. This means that these diets are destined to fail from the outset. Let's not fool ourselves, you *will* eventually succumb to temptation and eat the forbidden fruit (which is very unlikely to actually be 'fruit'!). The very strictness of these types of diets makes this outcome inevitable (we will cover our ability to exert willpower later in the book but for now you're going to have to take my word for this). The result is that you will either binge on these forbidden foods or you will feel like a failure and fall off the diet. The likelihood is that you'll do both. Either way, the diet is now definitely out of the window.

Putting you back in control

The good news is that the 3F System gives you control over the food you eat so it won't interfere with the way you live your life. Of course there are *some* rules but these are nice rules and I won't make you feel guilty if you 'forget' about them sometimes. I have isolated the more prescriptive parts of the 3F System to those meals consumed in the morning and early afternoon. Why is this? Because these are the times you are most likely to be busy. For a lot of us the mornings and early afternoons are spent rushing around getting from one place to another. At these times you can do without the hassle of deciding what you can or can't eat. Your food choices need to be easy. I have therefore helped you with this decision. If you stick with my suggestions you will have variety *and* lose fat.

Do you want to eat or do some maths?

Another failure of most diet systems is the over-reliance on either calorie counting or some other form of tracking the nutrients you're putting into your body. I've covered calorie counting before so you know my views on this aspect. The very fact that you're tracking whatever it is can, in my view, lead to obsessive behaviour. This can in turn lead to disorderly eating habits. Eating isn't about mathematics. It should be fun! Very many diets pitch themselves as far away from fun as you can possibly get. The 3F System has been designed to remove all counting and tracking from your diet. There are a few simple things you need to be aware of but nobody is going to give you an app to install to measure how 'good' you're being.

Why 'a little and often' doesn't work

I've broken down the principles of the 3F System into the main meals of the day and will explain the rationale for each stage as we go through. This isn't a diet that encourages you to take multiple small meals. There's a lot of talk about splitting your daily calorie intake into 5 or 6 small meals eaten at specific intervals. The theory is that you'll burn off whatever you've ingested before the next small meal and you'll keep your metabolism ticking over and therefore lose fat. In practice however the theory tends to fall down.

Let's assume you're on the go, rushing somewhere and you need to eat because it's exactly 3 hours since your last small meal. You find a shop selling fresh sandwiches. You enter the shop and are faced with a selection of choices. Here lies the problem – which one of these choices contains the 317 calories you need for this meal? Very few sandwiches will be under your target calorific intake. It's likely the majority of sandwiches will contain far more calories than you are 'allowed'. The result is that you will unwittingly over-eat for this meal. It's also very unlikely that you will compensate for this by consuming fewer calories at your next small meal.

Without proper and methodical planning (it's those strict rules again!) it's incredibly difficult for anyone to avoid over-eating when consuming several small meals a day. Instead of eating less food it's likely you'll eat more food. In addition, the food you consume will probably be of a lower nutritional value than if you'd just stuck to three main meals. Simply put, lots of small meals tend to become lots of slightly larger meals that will result in over-eating.

But what happens if you are confident that you will be able to properly plan and record your meals? Well, it's not good news. A number of studies conducted in both the UK and US have found that increasing meal frequency does *not* result in greater weight loss or fat burning compared to eating meals at normal intervals[14]. In fact one study concluded that consuming smaller and more frequent meals might actually increase hunger and the desire to eat[15]. So why go through all that hassle in the first place?

Lastly, there is also a social downside to eating frequent small meals. Human beings are social animals. We thrive on family and friends. What happens when your diet prevents you from eating with your family or enjoying a meal out with friends? Do you sit down at the restaurant and order two starters – one for now and one for in 3 hours time? Awkward! Such diets simply don't appreciate the reality of people's lives. This is why I developed the 3F System: to fit into the way you live your life.

Good things are worth waiting for

The aim of the 3F System is to provide a blueprint for healthy eating that will lead to sustainable fat loss. This is not a quick fix yo-yo diet. Before you start you need to 'buy in' to this being something that you will achieve over the medium to long term. This is because rapid fat loss is invariably followed by rapid fat *gain*. That said, you will certainly begin to feel the benefits of the 3F System almost immediately and will begin losing fat by following the simple programme within these pages. The ultimate aim is to alter your relationship with food so that you can lose fat and become healthier without the need to starve yourself or obsess about the things you want to eat.

Fix, Fuel & Fill for success

As mentioned at the beginning of this section, at the heart of the Final Countdown Diet is an approach to eating called the 3F System. The 3 Fs stand for 'Fix, Fuel & Fill'. The 3F System will guide all your main meal food choices. It's there for you when you're eating out and it's there for when you are cooking at home. Backing up the 3F System is advice for those occasions when you need to depart from the plan. The more perceptive amongst you will have realised that it's highly unlikely that the 3F System is going to be based around 5 or 6 small meals.

Instead I have concentrated on the three main meals of the day, which I have ingeniously called 'Breakfast, Lunch & Dinner'. However before we consider how to approach each of these main meals it's time to get an overview of the 'Fix, Fuel and Fill' system.

.

INTRODUCING THE 3F SYSTEM

In this section we introduce the 3F System. It is this system that is the bedrock of the Final Countdown Diet. It is this system that will govern what you put on your plate when you're preparing your main meals. It is this system that will help you on all those social occasions where you need to make a healthy food choice. It is this system that will ensure you can eat healthily whilst losing fat at the same time.

In line with the general theme of the Final Countdown Diet there are no 'banned' foods. There are however some foods that you should not consume in large quantities. These are typically foods that have high carbohydrate densities. When you eat such foods you are not only making it difficult for your body to process them, you are also loading your body with sugars that are likely to end up as fat.

The 3F System isn't however a low carb diet. I firmly believe that you need carbs and you shouldn't severely restrict them. I believe the 'trick' is to only consume as much energy as your body needs. How then does the 3F system work?

To make the 3F System workable in most situations I want you to imagine your plate is divided into three sections. The best way to do this is to draw an imaginary line down the middle of your plate. This will give you 2 halves. You then need to take one of these halves and further divide it into two. This will give you your three sections: two quarters and one half. These sections have been named Fix, Fuel and Fill and are the '3Fs' in the 3F System.

We are going to put specific types of food within in each section. The foods we put into each section have been designed to provide a nutritionally balanced diet that will both keep you healthy and also help you to lose body fat. The next few chapters will explain the 3F System in much more detail and will also provide guidance on the practicalities of fitting the 3F System into your daily life.

THE FIRST QUARTER: FIX

The first quarter of the plate is reserved for proteins. Proteins are there to help your body to develop and grow. They give your skin a healthy glow and make your hair shiny. When you are injured they assist with your recovery. They are your body's First Aid kit; this is why this section of the plate is called 'Fix'.

Where to find your protein fix

What do you put in this quarter? There are numerous sources of protein however the most readily available comes from meat, fish, poultry or eggs. If you are a vegetarian good sources of protein can be found in tofu, soya beans, nuts or legumes. In choosing your protein source try to avoid any heavily processed foods such as pies or ready meals.

If I were to create a league table of the best things to add to the Fix Section I would suggest that chicken would be at the top of the table. It's convenient, can be added to a whole range of dishes and is a good source of lean protein.

Something fishy

White fish such as Cod, Haddock, Plaice and Coley are also high up on the league table as they are lean and provide a decent source of Omega 3 fatty acids -which may help prevent heart disease. Oily fishes such as Salmon, mackerel, sardines, trout, fresh tuna and herring are also good sources of Omega 3 fatty acids although you should limit your intake of oily fish to a couple of occasions a week. This is because some oily fish contain low levels of pollutants that can build up in the body over time.

What about red meats?

Near the bottom of the league table are red meats such as beef, lamb and pork. However this is not because they are low in protein. On the contrary, beef in particular has high levels of protein. They are lower down because it is wise to limit consumption of red meat for a variety of health-related reasons. The trick is, as ever, to have a varied diet and don't overdose on any particular kind of meat. Limited quantities of red meat are fine. If you can, try to avoid any processed meats such as sausages, burgers, bacon and meat in pies etc. If you can't live without a burger why not make your own? I guarantee it'll be healthier and more satisfying than anything you'll find on a supermarket shelf.

Change the way you think about meat

Restricting protein to only one quarter of the plate may go against the grain. If you're anything like me then you were raised thinking that meat was the default centrepiece of any meal. Glorious Sunday Roasts spring to mind, as well as holidays such as Christmas and Thanksgiving that were centred around feasts of meat! The notion that you should reserve just a quarter of a plate for protein may therefore seem unusual. The fact is however that we tend to eat too much meat.

Our bodies obviously need protein but too much of it is derived from meat. This can have all sorts of effects on our bodies such as the formation of painful kidney stones, bowel complications and suchlike. Incidentally, the Chinese tend to eat meat as an accompaniment to a meal, not as the main ingredient. They add meat to provide flavour to their dishes and I think it works perfectly. Whichever way you choose to cook it, meat should only form a quarter of your plate.

Play your cards right

What you can't do however is create a 'meat mountain' on your plate and carefully trim the edges so they fit neatly within a quarter. Similarly you shouldn't go out and buy the largest plates known to man. That won't work. You need to stick to a normal plate and a defined portion size. For meat, that portion should be about the same size and height as a pack of playing cards. Whenever you are serving up or putting food on your plate visualise a pack of cards and stick to a similar sized quantity of meat. For fish, your portion size should be about the same size and thickness as the palm of your hand.

IN A NUTSHELL

- The 'Fix' Section is a quarter of a normal sized serving plate.
- Proteins belong in the Fix section. You can get proteins from meat, poultry, fish, eggs or from other sources such as legumes, tofu and quinoa.
- Try to avoid processed forms of protein as much as possible.
- A portion size of protein is the same size as a pack of cards for meat and the same size as the palm of your hands for fish.

THE SECOND QUARTER: FUEL

The second quarter of the plate is where you find the carbohydrates. Carbs have had a bad press recently. Low or No carb diets have become increasingly popular but also come with a health warning. They can effect your digestion, cause constipation and even result in kidney damage and other serious complications. The fact is you can't live without carbs or the energy they provide.

You need fuel for the journey

If you are lacking in energy then the chances are you are also lacking in carbs. You may well have tried a low carb diet in the past. If you did, it's likely that at some point you felt sluggish and had cravings for sugary things. You need carbs; they're the fuel tank in your body. This is why this section of our plate is named 'Fuel'. Foods in this quarter cover the whole spectrum from grains, legumes, pulses, pasta and vegetables so there are plenty of choices. As a guide, the below are some of the foods that would sit within the Fuel section:

Vegetables:

Potatoes
Parsnips
Peas
Pumpkin
Sweet Potatoes
Butternut Squash
Corn on the cob or sweetcorn

Grains / Legumes / Pulses:

Rice (brown rice is better than white rice)
Pasta & Spaghetti (wholegrain preferred)
Noodles
Cous Cous
Quinoa
Bulgar Wheat
Chickpeas
Hummus
Butter Beans
Cannellini Beans
Kidney Beans
Lentils

Dairy:

Cheese

A whole new ball game

The trick is to enjoy your carbs whenever they occur in your diet during the week but don't make them the mainstay of your menu. Keep them to their quarter and you'll be receiving just the right level of carbs to keep you healthy and moving about. Legumes such as Butter Beans and Lentils also provide a good source of protein and fibre. Fibre helps to slow down the absorption of any sugars.

How many of these carbs do you need to put on your plate? As a visual guide you're looking at a lump of food about the size of a tennis ball (but obviously flattened down a bit so it doesn't roll off the plate!). As an example, this might be a small cup of cooked rice, half a can of chickpeas or a good old dollop of mashed potato.

THE REMAINING HALF: FILL

The remaining half of the plate is reserved for those vegetables that are not high in carbs. Everyone knows that vegetables are good for you but we rarely eat enough of them. The government tells us to eat '5-a-day' but why are vegetables so important?

Vegetables are important because diets rich in vegetables may reduce heart disease. There is also evidence that they might protect against certain types of cancer and can reduce the risk of other ailments such as Type 2 Diabetes. Put simply vegetables help to ward off all the nasty things that might send us to an early grave.

However the benefits of vegetables don't end there. Not only are vegetables good for you, you can also eat loads of them without putting on a whole load of fat.

That's right. You can fill yourself up on vegetables with no or minimal impact to your fat levels. Can you guess the name of this part of the plate? You're right, it's the 'Fill' section!

Fill your plate

This section can be filled with great foods such as broccoli, fine beans, pak choi and salad vegetables such as cucumber, tomatoes and red peppers. There's a lot of good food in there and you can create some great dishes using this half. Below is just a selection of foods available via a major supermarket's website that would fit in the Fill section:

Vegetables:

Asparagus
Avocado
Aubergines/Eggplant
Beansprouts
Brocolli
Beetroot
Cabbage
Carrots
Cauliflower
Celeriac
Courgette/Zucchini
Fennel
Fine beans
Jerusalem Artichoke

Kale

Leeks

Lettuce

Mangetout

Marrow

Mushrooms

Okra

Olives - green and black

Onions

Pak choi

Radish

Red, yellow, green peppers

Rocket

Runner beans

Samphire

Salad vegetables (celery, cucumber, lettuce etc.)

Spinach

Spring onions

Sprouts

Swede

Tomatoes

Turnips

Watercress

It's another load of balls

Eating a variety of foods is highly beneficial so don't restrict yourself to just one choice of food for the Fill Section. Try to incorporate *at least* two varieties of vegetable to increase the benefit. For example, if you're creating a salad why not add shredded carrots, sliced tomatoes and chopped mushrooms to your salad vegetables? This gives you access to a whole host of different nutrients. As a simple rule of thumb, the more colours you have on your plate the wider the range of nutrients your food will have.

So what portion size are we looking at? As a minimum to give the body the nutrients it needs you're looking at two tennis balls. That said, this is the section of the plate you can be most generous with portion size. If you just *know* that two tennis balls is not going to be enough to fill you up until your next meal then please give yourself the serving size you deserve!

MAKING THE 3F SYSTEM WORK IN PRACTICE

Having now been given an overview of the 3F system you will be aware that we need to divide our plate into 3 sections. The first half of the plate is filled with proteins and starchy carbohydrates and the second half contains non-starchy vegetables. It's now worth considering an example of how this system would work in practice. Let's go back to my favourite pastime: Chinese Food!

I adore Chinese food and a typical Chinese restaurant meal will inevitably come with rice. Following the 3F System I understand that white rice has a high level of carbohydrates and therefore shouldn't form the mainstay of my meal. This gives me a few choices.

The first choice is to choose brown rice instead of white rice. Brown rice is full of fibre. This means that its sugars will be released more slowly compared to white rice. However, I find brown rice a bit of a chore to eat and I want to enjoy my food. In addition I've never been to a Chinese restaurant that serves brown rice so I guess that option is totally out.

My second option is to forget about rice altogether and choose something else. However that's not going to happen because I'm an adult and I want to eat rice! In addition, I also know that if I deny myself something my willpower will inevitably cave in and I'll end up eating it anyway. So what it the third option?

The third option is actually the preferred option. What I do is stick to the 3F System and I get myself a small bowl of rice. I make sure I only put a tennis-ball-sized lump on my plate and in that way I have now provided the Fuel Section of my plate. I can now turn my attention to filling the remaining sections.

I can easily find something to put in the Fix Section and in this instance I choose some stir fried chicken and peanuts. This provides a great source of protein and if I'm sharing the dish with friends the serving size shouldn't be too large. No matter, whatever sized serving I'm presented with I need to ensure that the Fix section only takes up a quarter of the plate. If I start feeling guilty about wasting food I can always take out a 'doggy bag' and save the food for a later meal. All I need to do now is order a vegetable dish or two to make up the rest of the plate.

Knowing Chinese food there's a great range of really tasty vegetables on offer. In this instance I choose steamed Pak Choi and also a fried aubergine (eggplant) dish. I find this is a great way to sample flavours and dishes that I may not have ordinarily chosen. It's certainly better than just sticking to meat and rice. By following the Fix, Fuel & Fill method I have instantly created a healthier Chinese meal than I've ever eaten before. What's more, I did this without having to memorise an excessive list of 'good' and 'bad' foods and without a calorie calculator in sight. But what happens if you want more?

The 3F System has been designed to give you the flexibility to create satisfying meals. Foods that are not only nutritionally balanced but also keep you feeling full. You may however find that sometimes you still feel hungry after your meal. If this happens then you should wait at least 20 minutes before considering a second helping. This will give your brain time to realise that you've had a satisfying meal and are actually full. If, after 20 minutes, you still feel hungry then choose a second helping – but choose it from the Fill section only.

The above is really what healthy eating is all about. It's about variety, careful selection of foods and not 'overdosing' on the things that will get you fat. It's as simple as that and the fresher the food – the better it is for you. The next section will focus on those in-between meal occasions when you need a drink or a snack to keep you going.

IN A NUTSHELL

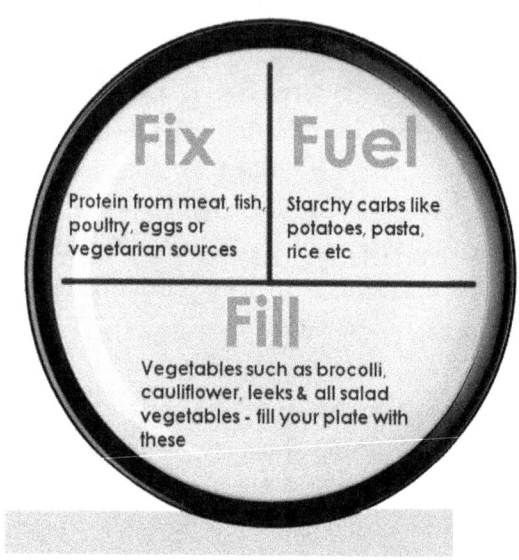

- The first quarter of the plate is the Fix Section. It contains the protein that helps your body rejuvenate itself. Your most likely source of protein will come from meat, fish or vegetarian options such as Tofu.

- The second quarter of the plate is the Fuel Section. This provides the drive and energy to get yourself through the day. This quarter exclusively contains foods that have moderate to high carbohydrate levels. Carbohydrates should not be the mainstay of your meal.

- The third and fourth quarters – the Second Half of the plate – contain the Fill section. This is loaded with foods that are beneficial to our health. This half is the domain of the vegetable. You need to see a lot of green in this section. It is this section that allows you to add more than the recommended serving size so the resultant meal is pleasantly filling.

- If you use a sauce try to ensure that its ingredients come exclusively from the Fill section of the plate without over-use of sugars, cream or other fats. Home-made is best.

- After you've eaten your meal allow at least 20 minutes before considering any second helpings.

DRINKS

There are three main drinks that I'm going to encourage you to drink whilst following the Final Countdown Diet. Each one of these drinks has health benefits although the benefits of some may not seem some obvious at first. Let's get the easy one out of the way first. Water!

Water

We all know how beneficial water is to our health. It keeps us hydrated and helps us to feel nice and full when our tummy is rumbling and pretending that it needs to be fed. But honestly, how many of us drink enough water throughout the day? As a guide a healthy adult will need to consume between 1.5litres and 2litres of water a day. This doesn't have to be just water itself. It's OK to drink this in coffee and tea, but water is obviously better for quenching your thirst. Just try not to mix it with anything that will add sugar: such as a fruit squash or cordial.

It might help for you to carry a 1ltr bottle of water around with you to drink as you go about your day. I put a bottle next to my laptop and whenever I'm reading through something on the screen I often find myself taking a swig of water without really thinking about it. The 1ltr bottle combined with other sources of water – such as tea and coffee – should be enough to keep you adequately hydrated. As a simple rule of thumb, if you go to the toilet and your urine is brownish, dark orange or dark yellow then you need to drink more water. If it's light yellow or clear - then good for you!

Just your cup of Tea

There are a variety of teas that will help you to achieve your fat loss goals. You may have heard about the wonderful benefits of Green Tea but did you know that Black Tea is also good for you?

Black Teas are those teas typically consumed in the UK and USA. These teas include standard varieties such as Assam or normal Breakfast Teas (or indeed Builders Tea!). Studies conducted in Japan seem to suggest that certain components, called polyphenols, that are found within black tea might prevent obesity by reducing the amount of fat absorbed by the body[16]. It is thought that the fat-fighting compounds are boosted when the tea leaves undergo fermentation – the process which turns the tea black.

It's important to say that to gain the maximum benefit you need to be drinking your tea without milk. We will talk later about the potential downsides of drinking lots of milk but there is another reason why it's not recommended to drink milky tea. Tea contains certain compounds called theaflavins and thearubigins which have been shown to prevent obesity in various scientific studies. However research conducted by scientists in India has shown that when you add milk to tea, these fat-fighting compounds are neutralised[17]. Put simply, the proteins found in milk stop the tea from fighting fat.

Go easy on the milk

I stopped drinking milk in tea ages ago. If you can't live without a milky cup of tea then the first thing you need to realise is that you absolutely and positively *can* live without a cup of milky tea. You just have to train your tastebuds. Did you know that your taste buds renew themselves every fortnight? It's true, they do. Therefore, to re-train your taste buds all you need to do is gradually reduce the amount of milk in your tea over a two-week period until you end up using no milk at all. Failing that you can go 'cold turkey' and start drinking tea without milk immediately. If you go cold turkey then you start receiving the benefits straight away although it might take some time for you to get used to the taste – but get used to the taste you will.

Going Green

Now on to our second tea option: Green Tea. This is the Daddy of the bunch when it comes to healthy tea options. We mentioned earlier that fermented black tea inhibits the absorption of fat into the body. Green Tea is thought to work in a different way.

Green Tea contains substances called 'catechins' which work as anti-oxidants. Green Tea also contains caffeine. It is believed that this caffeine and catechin mixture helps to increase the amount of energy your body burns. This has two distinct advantages. Firstly it means that any food you consume will be burnt off more rapidly with less chance of it getting stored as fat. Secondly, if your metabolism starts to slow down because you are losing weight then the increased energy burn from Green Tea will ensure your body keeps burning fat[18].

It gets better, once you've lost your fat and you continue to drink green tea there is evidence to show that the green tea catechins help to keep you at your new size[19]. In short, you need to introduce Green Tea into your life.

All the tea in China

There are many ways to start consuming Green Tea. A very simple way is to buy a pack of Green Teabags from the supermarket (most supermarkets stock Green Tea these days) and just add hot water as normal (no milk) and enjoy! I tend not to buy the teabags and instead get the loose tea leaves from a Chinese Supermarket. This is purely personal preference and has no impact on the benefits of the tea.

Wake up and smell the Coffee!

I love coffee. I can't get through the morning without a coffee and there's no reason why you should exclude coffee from your diet. As you are no doubt aware coffee contains caffeine. A low to moderate dose of caffeine will give you increased alertness, energy and a heightened ability to concentrate[20]. What is a low to moderate dose? About one cup of coffee (or two cups of green tea). So, coffee is a great way to achieve a decent dose of caffeine without drinking too much. You do however have to take this coffee black without sugar. By now you will understand that the combination of milk and/or sugar will not help you to lose fat. We therefore need to cut these out of our diets wherever we can.

Will drinking coffee on its own help you lose fat? It has to be said that the jury is out on that question. There has been some research on the effects that caffeine can have on weight loss. It has been suggested that caffeine helps you burn energy more quickly (thermogenesis) or that it helps to burn fat. Most of this research however has been done with a combination of green tea and caffeine and hasn't really included coffee in the mix.

Other research has shown that caffeine can help increase endurance and fat burning when undertaking exercise. If you are healthy and regularly exercise then it would do you no harm to take a cup of coffee about 90 minutes prior to your workout to take advantage of this effect. Coffee itself though is not proven to be as effective as Green or Black tea for fat loss purposes.

Sweet talk

Carbonated drinks tend to contain very high levels of sugars or sugars that are 'hidden' such as fructose. If you opt for the diet/lite version of a drink then be mindful that some research has shown that even these diet/lite options might lead to weight gain. Some scientists think that the sweeteners in the drinks actually trick your brain into thinking you are ingesting sugar with the result that your body starts storing this 'fake' sugar as fat. The theory is that when your brain gets a signal that you are eating something sweet it reacts in the same way it's always done and sets off the 'I'm eating sugar' mechanisms. The sweeteners seem to confuse your body's evolutionary responses[21]. We're back to the caveman/woman thing and your body's biology. But what does this mean in reality?

If I'm going to be totally honest I would say when faced between a choice between a diet and standard soft drink you should always go for the diet option. You know the standard version will contain an obscene amount of sugar so the damage it does to your body will be inevitable. The science surrounding the body's responses to the 'fake' sugar is less well developed so you might as well take a chance on the diet/lite option and hope it will pass through your body 'unnoticed'.

Juicy information

The received wisdom is that fruit juice forms part of your 5-a-Day and should be incorporated into your diet. I disagree. Here's why. Fruit juice admittedly tastes great but this is mainly because it's loaded with sugars: fructose to be precise. Drinking a glass of juice is different from eating the fruit it's made from. If you eat a piece of fruit you will consume a whole host of nutrients in addition to a good dose of fibre. We've spoken about fibre before. It's good for you because it slows down the way sugar is absorbed into your body. However, when a fruit gets processed into juice all of this fibre gets discarded as 'pulp' and dumped into a wheelie bin at the back of a factory somewhere. This leaves you with a drink laden with sugars but missing the very thing that will slow down their absorption. This sugar hits your body all at once and a large proportion of it will most likely get stored as fat. This is why you should avoid fruit juice.

Alcohol problem? What problem?

It might be pushing it too far if I suggest that alcohol will help you lose weight. Unfortunately it won't. Alcohol in its various forms typically contains lots of sugar without any nutritional value. However we are grown ups and the Final Countdown Diet is not designed to turn you into a hermit or to take you away from the things you enjoy. You may find yourself having a drink in a social situation or you may well want to crack open a bottle of wine after a hard day at work – and why not?

The trick is to choose your tipple carefully and stick to an acceptable volume. In terms of what's good to drink, I would suggest that a glass or two of red wine every so often wouldn't make much difference in the overall scheme of things. If you exceed this amount then you're not doing your body much good and you'll end up interfering with the way your body burns fat.

White wines tend to be sweeter and therefore contain more sugar so the intake of these should be restricted. The same is true of beers and lagers (there's a reason it's called a beer belly!). If you have to have a beer then opt for a 'lite' version. You should try to avoid cocktails as invariably they are made with fruit juices (see above) or sodas that are not the diet or lite version (also see above). If you absolutely have to have a cocktail – pick something that's made with a diet soda or soda water.

IN A NUTSHELL

- Water is not only the best thirst-quenching drink in the Universe, it's also brilliant at staving off false hunger pangs
- Green and Black Tea – taken without milk – can help you lose fat.
- Black Coffee might help in fat loss due to its caffeine content

- If you choose a carbonated drink try to make it a diet or lite option although some research suggests your body still thinks it's drinking the full sugar variety.
- Fruit juice – all the sugar and none of the goodness. Avoid!
- Alcohol – the rule of thumb is consume alcohol in moderation (but you knew that didn't you?)

SNACKS

The aim of the 3F System is to prevent you from feeling the need to snack. However I appreciate that sometimes you have a hunger pang that just won't go away. These hunger pangs will typically arrive in the late afternoon or some time after you've eaten in the evening. Drinking water, as previously discussed, can help overcome such pangs and it is to water that you should turn as a first resort. If you definitely can't survive without a snack then you need to find something to eat that has a high protein content. Many things that are traditionally regarded as snack foods, such as bags of crisps etc., are simply not going to keep you full and satisfied until the next meal.

Let's go Nuts!

In finding a high protein snack there are a range of choices. One good option is a handful of nuts. Almonds, hazelnuts or peanuts are preferable. A 'handful' is about the size of a golf ball. Almonds are particularly good for providing calcium. Peanuts are full of protein and fibre and will help you feel fuller for longer. Hazelnuts are rich in heart-friendly monounsaturated fats, Vitamin E and lots of good stuff like fibre, calcium, magnesium, zinc, folic acid and biotin. If you opt for a handful of nuts, you should choose a roasted and unsalted version.

Fill up with yoghurt

Another good snack option is yoghurt with high-protein content. Choose plain yoghurt over a flavoured option. The latter will invariably contain a lot of sugar. In a study conducted to discover the benefits of a high-protein snack versus a snack with high fat levels[22] (they used crackers and chocolate) it was found that yoghurt helped keep the participants fuller for longer. Interestingly, the participants also ate fewer calories during the evening meal than they would if they had eaten the high fat snack. The study concluded that snacks such as high-protein yoghurt help to improve appetite control, help to keep you full and will reduce the amount you eat at later meals.

Don't get fruity

What about fruit? I'm not a big fan of snacking on fruit - or eating fruit per se. This is why fruit is barely mentioned within this book. The problem with fruit is that people often turn to it as a healthy option when they're hungry. The more you eat the healthier you'll get! However depending on which fruit you choose this 'healthy' snack might actually be filling you up with sugar. We spoke earlier about fruits being high in fructose. We know from earlier discussions that anything ending in 'ose' is basically a sugar. An overload of sugar will end up being stored in your fat cells. The more fruit you eat the more likely this is to happen. Some fruits contain fibre - which is good for slowing down the release of sugars - but this will only work on relatively low levels of sugar. To keep sugar intake at a low level the best option is the humble apple. Apples contain a significant amount of fibre, are vitamin and mineral rich and are also easy to carry around. You don't even have to peel them. Bonus!

Chocoholics Delight!

Here's one to put a smile on your face. Chocolate! Yes, Chocolate is OK but there is a caveat to this - only Dark Chocolate and only in small quantities. What do I mean by Dark Chocolate? I mean high cocoa content chocolate – typically containing in excess of 70% cocoa. What do I mean by small? Unfortunately small in this instance is just a square of chocolate and I would limit this to 2 or 3 times a week. It may be enough to satisfy any chocolate cravings but it certainly won't fill you up and stave off any hunger.

The reason chocolate is allowed is that dark chocolate in particular contains polyphenols and flavanols. These compounds have been shown to reduce risk factors for Type 2 diabetes and certain heart diseases. There are also some scientific studies that suggest consuming dark chocolate in moderation may help to reduce the body's absorption of fats and carbohydrates[23].

IN A NUTSHELL

- Go nuts for nuts! A handful of nuts contains a good amount of protein that will keep you feeling full. Stick to unsalted versions.

- Yoghurt with high protein content has been proven to keep you feeling fuller for longer and might help you to eat less at later meals.

- Try to not get hung up on eating fruit and kidding yourself it's going to help you lose fat. Fruit contains sugars. If you must eat fruit, try an apple.

- Chocolate! What's not to love? Choose the high cocoa content varieties and eat only in small quantities. It won't fill you up but it's got some real health benefits.

BREAKFAST AND LUNCH

The Fix, Fuel & Fill system can be applied to all mealtimes. Think of a cooked breakfast with a couple of poached eggs forming the Fix section. A portion of baked beans or fried potatoes providing the Fuel and some lovely griddled tomatoes and mushrooms making up the Fill section. Yummy! However let's face it, how many of us get up in the morning and have the *time* to cook breakfast? For this reason it's useful to have other 'weapons' in your armoury that will ensure you can continue with your fat loss aims.

This chapter looks at breakfast and lunch times. These are the occasions when you are most likely to be rushing about and eating on the go. Although you will still want to eat healthily at these times, your ability to follow the 3F System may be limited. What follows therefore are some suggestions for your breakfasts and lunches. These suggestions will ensure you maintain a balanced diet whilst helping you to lose fat at the same time.

BREAKFAST

Breakfast - the most important meal of the day! You will have heard this so many times that it's probably become boring to hear. Some diets however suggest that you ignore breakfast entirely. The rationale for this is that if you skip breakfast you will save calories. However as we have seen in earlier chapters - it isn't that simple. The result of force-starving yourself is that your body starts to hold on to all those resources it needs to keep you alive. Specifically it holds onto those little bundles of energy it keeps in your fat cells. Skipping breakfast *per se* is therefore not a good idea.

Other diets take the opposite approach and tell you that you *must* eat breakfast precisely because it is *so* important. Some even prescribe that you need to eat it within a certain timeframe of waking to get the full benefit. These diets are pretty prescriptive and don't seem to 'get' how people actually live.

Eat when you need to

The FCD Plan takes a simpler and less prescriptive approach to breakfast. My view is that you *should* eat breakfast – but only when you *feel* like you need to. Let me explain. The time I eat breakfast tends to vary from day to day. Sometimes I'm tucking into breakfast at 07:30. The day of writing this I ate at 09:45. Generally though I start feeling a bit hungry just before mid-morning and *that's* when I have my breakfast. This is when my body tells me I need to eat. This point is key.

You need to listen to your body and you need to differentiate between the *need* to eat and the *desire* to eat. The 'need' to eat is when your body tells you you're hungry. It is a biological function and it is your body signaling to you that you'd better find it some energy quick. The 'desire' to eat is more emotional and can be caused by many factors – not least by how tempting that piece of cake looks! How can you tell between the need to eat and the desire to eat?

'Need' and 'Desire' are not the same

The *need* to eat is caused by your body telling you you're hungry. You have that feeling of hunger. When you feel this, a good tool is to absorb yourself in doing something else to distract the craving. Also grab yourself a glass or two of water to see if that helps. If it doesn't go away or increases over time then this is definitely the need to eat.

The *desire* to eat on the other hand does not produce the same feeling of physical hunger. Many things can trigger the desire to eat. It might be caused by some emotional reaction, such as being stressed or upset, that can only be pacified by 'comfort food'. TV adverts can trigger the desire, as can a lovely aroma wafting out of a café window as you pass by. The initial response to the desire to eat is the same as with the need to eat. Attempt to distract the craving by doing something else. If the distraction makes the craving go away then it's purely an emotional desire and should be ignored.

Listen to your body

The key is to listen to your body and only eat breakfast when you feel hungry. If you're not feeling hungry then it's likely your body is still enjoying the previous night's meal and isn't yet ready to eat. The distraction methods mentioned earlier might seem odd but sometimes the reason we've put on fat in the first place is because we've spent too long listening to our desires and forgotten all about what it feels like to be hungry. Be honest, when was the last time you really, physically, felt hungry? So often we reach for a snack just because it's there and not because we physically need to eat.

This next point is however critical. For all the reasons mentioned earlier in this book - this is *not* about starvation. I am in no way suggesting you stretch out your hunger for a specific period or wait until the hunger is so crippling that you need to gorge on food to satisfy it. The aim of listening to your needs and desires is to identify exactly when you're body is ready to eat. Once you've identified this – you should eat when your body is ready.

Over time this will become second nature and you'll just *know* when the time is right to eat. You will have trained your brain to recognise that you need to eat and you won't need to employ any distraction techniques. Until that time however start slowly and start listening to your body. When you feel hungry try to distract yourself. Learn to recognise the differences in the way you feel between when you *need* to eat rather than when you have the *desire* to eat.

I've missed breakfast. What now?

What should you do if you've lasted the whole morning and not had breakfast because you've not felt hungry? First you need to understand that you've not felt hungry simply because you didn't need to eat. It's likely your body had enough energy stored up inside to cope with an extra few hours without taking more energy onboard. In such circumstances it's perfectly fine to have lunch as your first meal of the day and carry on from there. We've all skipped breakfast at some point in our lives and we're still here to tell the tale. If you do skip breakfast then you may feel hungry later on in the day. If this occurs then have a snack. Snacking options were covered earlier in the book.

BREAKFAST OPTIONS

This section of the book will consider the options for those times when you're simply too busy to fit the 3Fs into your breakfast routine. I will tell you the best, most satiating and most convenient options for breakfast. These options stick closely to the whole ethos of the 3F System. The aim is to provide protein, energy and also to keep you full. If you choose these options and stick with the Fix, Fuel and Fill system for the rest of your meals then you *will* lose fat. Read on to find out what breakfast looks like on The Final Countdown Diet.

If you look back on your breakfast habits over the past month my guess is you probably ate the same things over and over again with little variation. This is not unusual. Most of us have the same type of things for breakfast every morning. Our breakfasts are dictated by our tastes, our habits, our lifestyle or a combination of the above. The FCD Plan provides two choices for breakfast. These can be interchanged throughout the week to provide variety or to fit in with your lifestyle. Obviously you also have the option of following the Fix, Fuel & Fill system whenever circumstances dictate.

The suggested breakfast options have been chosen for a reason. In fact it's two reasons. They've been chosen because they help you to feel full and because they provide you with the energy you need to get through the morning. OK, there's a third reason, they're also backed up by scientific studies that highlight these choices as being beneficial for those wanting to lose fat.

Go to work on an egg

First on the menu is Eggs on Toast – with a twist. It's generally understood that you should limit your intake of bread because it is made from flour. Flour is 100% carbohydrate so it will transport sugar into your bloodstream. Too much sugar turns to fat. However, as this is the morning you will need energy, therefore toast is perfectly acceptable for this mealtime. There is however something special about this toast. To make this toast special you first need to use bread that has previously been frozen. This might sound like a hassle but in reality you won't be eating too much bread so it's actually a sensible way to stop waste and save you money. However the bread isn't frozen to save you money, it's frozen to help you lose fat.

Let's propose a toast

There is a thing called the Glycaemic Index ("GI") that you may well have heard of. The GI is basically a way of classifying how different foods raise the level of glucose (sugar) in your blood. It is generally accepted that eating foods that won't raise your blood sugar is good for you and some diet plans have been built around low GI foods. How then does this relate to your humble slice of toast?

A study conducted by researchers from Oxford Brookes University[24] in the UK found that when bread was frozen, defrosted, and toasted something happened to the GI level within the bread. It became lower. What this means is that the carbohydrates from *this* toast will be lower than normal and the energy will be released more slowly into your bloodstream. It is for this reason that you must freeze, defrost and toast your bread. This 'low GI' toast provides your Fuel Section however a slice or two of toast is unlikely to fill you up. This is where the eggs come in.

Eggs are great. They are nutrient dense and contain lots of vitamins and minerals, including calcium, which is vital for healthy teeth and bones. Eggs are also a magnificent source of protein. This is essential for the growth and repair of your body's cells and tissues. Eggs therefore provide the 'Fix' component to your breakfast. But the greatness of eggs doesn't end there.

Various studies have shown that eggs are ideal for those wanting to lose fat. In particular, eggs have been shown to promote 'satiety'. This means they help you to feel full so you don't need to eat more. In one study[25], overweight and obese participants were given either an egg breakfast or one consisting of an equally calorific intake of bagels. Those who ate eggs for breakfast felt fuller for longer and also ate significantly less in the short term. So, not only do eggs provide the Fix section, they also provide the Fill Section as well. Other studies[26] have shown that eating eggs for breakfast actually enhanced weight loss in overweight or obese subjects.

Your ideal breakfast on the Final Countdown Diet is therefore one or two slices of toast (from bread that's been previously frozen) accompanied by two eggs. The carbohydrate within the toast forms the Fuel Section and the eggs provide both the Fix and Fill Sections. What then is the best way to prepare your eggs?

To be honest, it doesn't really matter how you prepare the eggs. I like mine either boiled or poached but sometimes will opt to fry them. I like my eggs runny and I generally use the yolk to 'butter' my toast. If you're thinking of taking your breakfast to work – to eat once hunger sets in – then it's obviously better to have boiled eggs. If you do this then you can simply take your bread out of the freezer in the morning and let it defrost during the trip into work.

Eggs for the time-starved

Here's a quick breakfast solution if you need to eat in a hurry. First, pop the bread into the toaster. While it's toasting away, grab a mug and half-fill it with water. Crack an egg into the mug and put it into the microwave. Depending on your power setting you will need to cook it for 60-90 seconds. After a minute check that the egg is cooked properly and adjust the time if needed. If you're having two eggs, simply repeat the process. Serve the eggs on top of the toast. Instant poached eggs on toast! A bodybuilder taught me this supremely quick method of poaching eggs. One thing I learnt from the sports nutrition business is that if someone eats the same thing every day they become very efficient at food preparation!

Get your oats

I did promise you another healthy and nutritious breakfast component and here it is: oats! If you didn't give yourself an imaginary high-five when you read that last sentence you obviously don't know your oats. Let me tell you how good oats are.

Compared with most other breakfast cereals, oats are better at controlling appetite[27] and increasing satiety. This is because Oats contain beta-glucan, which has been found to help people feel fuller for longer. In a study of overweight people it was also shown that those who ate an oat-based meal ate less at subsequent meals[28].

Oats also have other nutritional benefits. They are a good supply of fibre and protein but are lower in sugar than many cereals. The sugars they do contain are released slowly into the bloodstream thereby giving you a nice and even release of energy without it going straight to your fat cells. Basically, oats are the 3F System in a bowl!

What's the best way to prepare your oats? I prefer to make mine with hot water instead of milk. This avoids taking in any unnecessary sugars from the lactose in milk. In the interests of making life easy I tend to ignore the instructions on the side of the box that say you should boil your oats in a pan of water. I simply put about 80g of oats into a bowl and add boiling water from the kettle and stir until mixed in. This is quicker than standing over a pan and leaves you with fewer pots to clear up. You may have noticed that I specifically stated that I use about 80g of oats. Portion size is important to understand.

Portion size is key

We've all seen the nutritional information plastered on the side of many cereal packets. What you may not have realised is that many of the serving sizes on popular cereals are based around a *child's* portion! This means that all the calories and the Guideline Daily Amounts related to that serving are all kiddie-sized. Scale up your portion to a normal adult-sized serving and suddenly the nutritional information doesn't seem so healthy. If you eat cereal on a regular basis then my guess is you are probably eating well in excess of the recommended serving size.

As an experiment I once watched my wife fill her bowl with Cornflakes. Once the bowl was filled I grabbed it and weighed out the Cornflakes. It's great fun living with me – as you can probably tell. On weighing the Cornflakes I discovered that Jane's serving size was *four* times the amount recommended on the side of the packet. Basically she was consuming 400% more calories and carbs than she realised.

For your oat breakfast try to aim for a serving size equivalent to 350-500 calories a bowl. I promise, this is the *only* time you need to count calories. It's here because there's no other way of consistently measuring different varieties of breakfast cereal. To get to your serving size you first need to calculate how many grams of oats will provide you with those 350-500 calories. The nutritional information on the side of the packet will give you a guide. Once you have this figure, you then need to weigh out the appropriate amount of oats directly into a bowl. To make things easier going forward you should use the same bowl every day and always fill it to the same level.

Variety is the spice of life

The recommended breakfasts should become part of your weekly routine – alternating as required to break things up a bit. I have chosen them because I believe they are the best options for a healthy and filling breakfast. What happens though when you get really bored of eating them? If that happens then give yourself a break. A bit of variety is perfectly fine.

All you need to do is stick with the 3F System principles when choosing your alternative breakfasts. A reasonable alternative that can be made quickly is Beans on Toast. If your toast is prepared from frozen bread and you use decent quality baked beans then you'll be getting all of the Fix, Fuel & Fill elements. Some high fibre cereals are also a good alternative to Oats but don't drown them in milk and measure out the serving sizes as detailed earlier. But what happens if you get tempted by more 'naughty' breakfasts?

It has to be said that there will be occasions when it is not possible to stick to the 3F System. For example, you may wake up one morning to find the Croissant Fairy has visited you in the night. If that happens then simply just get back on the plan the very next mealtime. Life is about variety and denying yourself something naughty for breakfast is not going to do you any favours. However, this is NOT a 'get out of jail' card!

If you constantly revert back to your old unhealthy

breakfasts then you'll get the same result you've always got. I find it helps if you start the day focusing on the overall goal of sustainable and permanent fat loss. Ask yourself two simple questions. How will I look in a year's time if I stick to the plan? How will I look if I fall off the plan today? Once you've arrived at your answer then hopefully it will make it easier for you to stay with the system for the rest of the day.

IN A NUTSHELL

- There is no set time to eat breakfast. If you are not hungry when you wake up then don't immediately have breakfast. Instead wait until you feel like you want to eat. If you don't want to eat in the morning, the first meal of the day will be your lunch.

- If the first meal of the day turns out to be lunch then you need to be mindful that you might need to snack later in the day to give you an energy boost.

- You can use the 3F System for your breakfasts or opt for the choices I recommend. These choices will keep you energised and full throughout the morning.

- Breakfast One: One or Two Eggs served with a slice or two of toasted bread that has previously been frozen

- Breakfast Two: Approximately 80g of Rolled Oats prepared with boiling water. Avoid "instant" or "simple" varieties as they contain sugars.

- If you fancy a break from the preferred breakfasts then you should bear in mind the Fix, Fuel & Fill

System.

LUNCH

This will most likely be your second meal of the day. By now you will have eaten breakfast when you first started to feel hungry and this breakfast will have kept you full for a good few hours. You've also had a couple of drinks of coffee, tea or water and, as a result, you should have felt pretty satiated throughout the course of the morning. So, what time are you going to sit down to eat your lunch? The answer is similar to that given for breakfast – when you start to feel hungry.

We discussed earlier the importance of recognising when our bodies are telling us we physically *need* to eat. We considered the difference between the need to eat and the desire to eat. Lunchtime is the second occasion of the day when we should be listening to what our bodies are telling us. On the FCD Plan you should not start to experience the *need* to eat until around 4 hours after you have eaten your breakfast.

Talk to your stomach

If you feel hungry prior to the 4-hour period elapsing then you should try to rationalise with your impulses. Say to yourself "I can't be hungry, I only ate two hours ago". Grab yourself a drink of coffee, tea or water to get something in your stomach to calm that urge down. I fully realise that this might seem easy to say and harder to put into practice but it is only by putting this into practice that you will get over these initial impulses. This is the first step to eating a more balanced and healthier diet – with the ultimate aim of losing fat.

Lunchtime is when you want it to be

With the above in mind you should try to avoid eating lunch at a set time every day. You want to avoid filling yourself full of energy your body doesn't need. In addition, watching the clock countdown to lunchtime can actually start your tummy rumbling and create false sensations of hunger. I attempt to avoid watching the clock and try to keep my lunchtime flexible. On some days I don't even start feeling hungry until 2pm – that time then becomes my lunchtime. I appreciate that your daily routine might not be as flexible so I've tried to keep the lunch options simple and easy thereby allowing you to prepare and eat them quickly.

Be mindful though, this is *not* an endurance test or a starvation diet. You don't get any points for stretching out the timeframe between breakfast and lunch to an unrealistic level. The aim is to simply eat when you actually, really, feel hungry. If you've followed the recommended breakfasts (or applied the 3F System) the timeframe between breakfast and lunch is likely to be around 4 hours. For myself, I find that if I've eaten at 07:30 I will start to feel hungry shortly before 12. This feeling invariably comes on suddenly and I make sure I get something to eat very shortly thereafter. I like to think I'm training my body to recognise that if it sends out false sensations of hunger then it's not going to be rewarded. If however it only sends me hunger signals when I am actually hungry it will be rewarded with a swift meal.

What a Souper idea!

What do I recommend for lunch? My recommendation is something that is easy to cook, easy to carry around and is nourishing. That 'something' is soup. Now you may love soup or you may loathe it but there are a few good reasons why you should make this your second meal of the day. The principal reason is that you'll lose fat if you follow my advice and have soup for lunch. If you eat what you've always eaten for lunch then the chances are you will not make much of a difference to your body size. Again this boils down to what's important to you. If losing fat – at this point in time – is important then you need to make some changes.

Convenience comes in cans

A clear benefit of soup is that it's convenient. Chances are that no matter what your daily routine is you can find a place for soup. If you spend your days at work then it's pretty easy to carry in a carton, a tin or a flask of soup to decant into a mug and heat in a microwave. It's quick, cheap, doesn't require a trip to the café down the road and is good for you. You may think that soup is uninspiring but the varieties and flavours available today make this a far from boring food choice. Soup is also incredibly easy to make at home.

Just like Mum used to make

When I'm at home I always try to make my own soup from fresh ingredients. The major benefit of this is that you know the quality and freshness of what you're putting into it. It actually *feels* like it's going to do you good. Making soup is simply a matter of simmering a few ingredients together and blasting them in a blender. It's as simple as that and there are lots of recipe books out there so you never need to get bored. You can also have hot soups in winter and cold soups in summer.

To make an easy task even easier I have invested in a Soup Maker. Using an electric soup maker is both convenient and cuts down on the washing up. You simply pop the ingredients into the soup maker, set the timer and sit back whilst the soup simmers away. Once done you blend it together and serve straight from the blender jug. However soup isn't included in the Final Countdown Diet purely because it's convenient and is a breeze to make; you should know me better than that!

Eat Soup. Get Slim

One major reason for including soup in your diet is because eating soup is associated with a lower risk of obesity: it's true. A study published in the British Journal of Nutrition[29] found that people who ate soup had a lower body weight and thinner waists than people who didn't tend to eat soup. Not only that, soup eaters ate more nutrients, vitamins and minerals when compared with non-soup eaters.

Other studies have also found that soup consumption is linked to a reduced risk of being overweight or obese[30]. Furthermore, studies from around the world seem to indicate that it doesn't matter where you live – if you eat soup – you're likely to be thinner. Here's one for you - in Japan it was found that there was an inverse association between the number of times you ate soup and waist circumference[31]. Put simply, people who eat soup frequently have thinner waists! Similar results have been found in European studies.

How does soup help us to lose weight? Several features of soup have been suggested as likely causes for weight loss. These features include the amount of soup consumed, the fat and energy content of the soup and even the form of the soup itself – basically whether it is thick, chunky or runny. However scientists have found no real difference between any of these features with regards to weight loss[32]. Basically no matter what type of soup you enjoy - you're going to feel full and lose weight.

The best starter in the world

Soup is also the best starter in the world. Fact! If you're out with friends and everyone is having a starter why should you sit out that course simply because you want to lose fat? Let's live in the real world - eating healthily is not about losing your friends! If soup is on the menu, have it as a starter. The scientists found that simply eating soup before the main course meant that people would consume fewer calories overall whilst actually eating more food in terms of weight. Just in case you weren't paying attention, the scientists found that soup as a starter allows a greater weight of food to be consumed with fewer calories compared with just going straight into a main meal. Believe me, soup is the way forward and that's why we have it as the main lunch for the FCD Plan.

Obviously for those times when soup is not on the menu, or you fancy a change, your fallback position is always going to be the 3F System. If you focus on including the Fix, Fuel & Fill elements into your eating you'll be both satisfied and will lose fat. With the Final Countdown Diet your healthy meal options are virtually limitless.

IN A NUTSHELL

- Eat lunch only when you start to feel hungry. Listen to your body. This doesn't have to be at everyone else's lunchtime.

- Soup is the best option for lunch. It's convenient, there are lots of varieties and you can easily create your own. It's also been found to help with weight loss.

- For all those other occasions when you are not having soup, your diet needs to incorporate the 3F System.

SEEDS, SAUCES & THINGS TO WATCH OUT FOR

THE SECRET SEED

What happens if you're following the FCD Plan and can't seem to satisfy your hunger? If it's genuine hunger and drinking water or consuming the snacks mentioned above won't satiate it then it's time to enlist our 'secret weapon': the Chia Seed. If you're unacquainted with these marvellous little black seeds, they originate from South America and can be used in a variety of foods. They're a good source of protein, contain loads of Omega 3, and the majority of the carbs come from fibre. The seeds also contain lots of other good things like zinc and calcium. But it's not for their nutritional benefit that you'll be primarily using them.

In addition to their nutritional value, Chia seeds having

another great quality; Chia Seeds swell up like crazy when added to liquid! If you do a search online you'll find some images of what happens when you add Chia seeds to water. Basically they grow into a gloop that looks a bit like frogspawn. Admittedly this doesn't immediately sound appetising but if you add a tablespoon of seeds to your breakfast cereal, salad, soup or whatever and keep your fluid intake up then the seeds will expand inside your stomach. This, combined with the protein and fibre content of the Chia Seed, will result in you feeling a lot fuller than you normally would. Your hunger pangs should then start to go away.

It's important though that you don't view Chia Seeds as the only solution. It has to be said that clinical trials on Chia Seeds are extremely limited. One study[33] found that overweight or obese adults did not experience any change in their body mass after Chia was consumed. It is not clear from the papers I have read whether or not the participants continued to consume their normal diet with Chia Seeds added. It stands to reason that if you continue to eat high volumes of unhealthy foods then the effect of the seeds on any weight loss will be minimised. However consumed within the context of The Final Countdown Diet they might just provide a useful tool to combat genuine hunger pangs.

A WORD ABOUT SAUCES

Nobody is expecting you to eat a dry plate of food. Some foods go exceptionally well with a sauce or gravy.

Some meals, such as curries, are completely based around the sauce. What we need to realise however is that sauces are not 'free'. Whilst a dash of soy sauce, a splash of olive oil or a balsamic dressing is unlikely to do you any harm, problems can arise when the sauce itself is the main component of the meal. If you tend to get your sauces out of a jar then you're likely to be consuming high amounts of sugar and other 'baddies'. You therefore need to carefully consider both your choice of sauce and the quantity you use.

Create your sauce from the Fill Section

Whenever possible you should make your own sauces. This way you can keep an eye on what's going into them. Most traditional sauces, such as tomato-based dishes, can be made solely from ingredients found in the Fill section of the plate. As long as the sauce isn't made with sugars or cream etc. there is no need to count it separately. Tomato based sauces can easily be knocked up with a can of tinned tomatoes or passata (check the ingredients don't contain high levels of salt or other baddies) along with a few herbs and spices. Which brings us on to spices.

Go spicy to burn fat

Spices make our foods burst with flavour. There is absolutely no need for the food you cook to be dull! I like a good curry and have found that it's relatively easy to make my own curry without opening a jar to do so. There are a multitude of curry recipes online and all you need to do is avoid those full of cream and yoghurt and opt for the tomato-based ones. You may well find that it tastes better than a curry in a jar and it will be better for you as well. What's more, the key component of chilli powder is capsaicin. This component has been shown to assist with weight loss in a number of ways. It is thought that eating capsaicin increases thermogenesis – the amount of energy your body burns. Capsaicin is also thought to deter fat cell growth and reduce food consumption[34]. So, make it spicy and start burning fat!

FOODS TO WATCH OUT FOR

Hopefully I've made it clear that the Final Countdown Diet Plan is not about banning the things you love to eat. I have though stressed that it's better to prepare foods yourself rather than rely on processed foods. Some foods however need to be consumed with caution – no matter who makes them. Such foods are typically very high in carbohydrates. The aim therefore is to restrict the amount that you eat of these foods. Think of this section not as a list of banned foods, but a list of foods you should be consume in moderation.

Keep off the white stuff

First on the list is flour. All flour – whether white, brown or wholemeal - is basically pure carbohydrate. Even though brown or wholemeal flour contains fibre, it is still about 76% carbohydrate. Where do you find flour? You know the culprits: bread, cakes and all sorts of things like bagels. Flour is also typically an ingredient in batters (such as for pancakes and Yorkshire puddings). Flour is also commonly used as a thickening for sauces (béchamel or roux sauce). Also be mindful of foodstuffs that might be coated or mixed with flour-based products – think fish or chicken in breadcrumbs. Your body simply can't process adequately the volume of carbohydrate found in flour-based products. If you're serious about losing fat you need to think seriously about restricting your intake of flour.

Let's talk Italian

Next on the list is pasta. Pasta is typically made from wheat flour. As with all other flour-based products, pasta is energy dense. If you eat pasta in moderation and keep it to the Fuel section of the plate then there's no problem. If however you make pasta the mainstay of every meal then you will be getting too much energy per meal and you will start to store that energy as fat. The aim is to keep your pasta to the Fuel Section of your plate and don't let it creep into other areas. As mentioned previously, take care over your choice of sauce and don't let any hidden sugars creep in.

Don't cry over spilled milk

The third thing you should limit is Milk. "What's wrong with good old milk?" I hear you say. Well firstly milk contains lactose. Those of you who were paying attention in the 'counting calories' chapter will remember that most foods with ingredients ending in 'ose' are full of hidden sugars. Milk is no exception to this rule. Milk contains a high volume of sugars and is used very effectively by bodybuilders to actually put on weight. Diet food it ain't.

You need to be careful about the volume of milk you consume on a daily basis. It is for this reason that milk wasn't included in the recommended Oats breakfast. However, if you can't live without milk in your cereal then it's an inevitable balancing act between the sugars in milk and the amount of fibre in your chosen cereal. The more fibre then the slower the absorption of the milk's sugars.

The main thing linking all of the above is that these foods are all relatively dense in carbohydrates. Another coincidental link is that all of these foodstuffs are white. As a rough and ready guide, if you're faced with a white carbohydrate then you need to be extra vigilant about keeping it to the Fuel section of your plate; it also shouldn't form the core of your daily diet.

IN A NUTSHELL

- If you limit certain foods your diet will be more effective
- Flour comes in many guises and you should educate yourself as to which foodstuffs contain flour
- Pasta is also energy dense. Keep it to the Fuel section of the plate and be careful you don't smother it in carb-heavy sauces.
- Milk contains sugars which will end up as fat. If you consume milk then try to offset this with a fibre-rich accompaniment.
- As a guide – be wary of white carbohydrates

WHAT ABOUT THE RECIPES?

Here's the thing about recipes in diet books. They limit your choices and they limit your options. Sure, they might provide inspiration but they also close off your mind to a whole range of foods that might actually be good for you. Recipes are basically another person's idea of what you want to eat. The 3F System is not about stopping you eating the foods you love (unless the foods you love are heavily processed and manufactured!). The 3F System is about placing the foods you eat in their rightful place on the plate and keeping the quantities at a reasonable and healthy level.

This is what your 3F plate looks like:

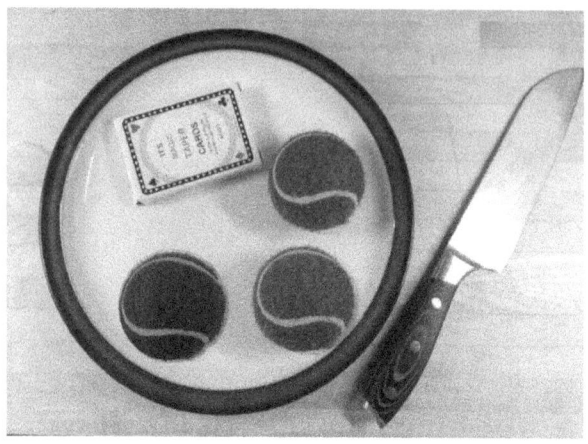

Sorry, I couldn't resist it (it seemed funny at the time). Anyway, back to the serious stuff. The *following* is an example of what a typical 3F plate should look like:

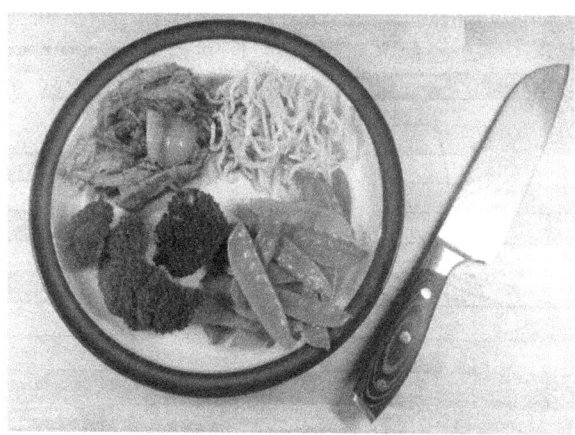

The meal in the above picture was cooked on the day I

wrote this section. It didn't need any special planning or a calorie calculator. All I did was look in the fridge, take out a few ingredients and assemble them following the 3F System. Let's take a closer look at the meal.

Fix

The meal itself is simple homemade sweet and sour pork with noodles, mange tout and broccoli. The pork provides the Fix section. This was left over from the previous day's meal (Pulled Pork – yummy!) so it was already cooked and just needed reheating. I made the sweet and sour sauce by simmering some chopped tomatoes (from a tin) in a pan until they reduced down a bit. Thereafter I added black vinegar and a dash of soy sauce. This made the sauce 'sour' with the natural sweetness of the tomatoes providing the 'sweet' element. I didn't use any sugar. I then heated through the pork in the pan and added some chopped pepper for a bit of colour and crunchiness.

Although the main element of the Fix section is protein, it's not a sin to 'borrow' a few vegetables or a simple sauce from the Fill section to make the meal more interesting. Remember, you can eat as much as you want from the Fill section so if your sauce is made entirely from Fill ingredients there's no harm.

Fuel

The Fuel section, the carbohydrate element, consisted

of the noodles. I soaked these in hot water until they were soft and then lightly tossed them in sesame oil to provide flavour and to stop them sticking. I didn't do anything else to cook them.

Fill

The Fill section, the vegetable element, was made up of broccoli and mange tout. Both of these were put in a steamer with the broccoli being given a few more minutes at the start to cook through. The Fill section contains more than two tennis balls of food however this is allowed in the 3F System. This is because Fill ingredients are nutritious and have low carbohydrate densities.

You will see from the photograph that the Fix and Fuel sections of the plate: the sweet and sour pork and the noodles - are pretty much bang on the size of a pack of cards and a tennis ball. Don't forget that the sauce was made exclusively from Fill ingredients. The quantity of pork itself is correct.

The whole meal, including the sauce, took about 15 minutes from start to finish. I hope this illustrates that you don't need recipes to follow the 3F System. Would it win an award at a Chinese Cookery Festival? Highly unlikely, but my family enjoyed it which is the main thing.

Whatever you might think about my cooking or my choice of food, the fact is that I did what a lot of people do on a daily basis. I went to the fridge, took out whatever was available, and then I cooked it. You may be a better cook than me. You may be a worse cook than me. It doesn't matter. Real food does not come in a container that you have to prick with a fork before putting it in the microwave. Real food is made using decent fresh ingredients - sometimes with the help of a tin of something that isn't loaded with additives. Real food doesn't have to be piled high on the plate to fill you up. Real food also doesn't have to be expensive. If you look again at the ingredients I used: leftover pork, a small portion of noodles, a tin of tomatoes and a bit of broccoli and mange tout – you'll find that the entire cost of the meal is much less than the cost of an average ready meal. What's more I made the dish for 5 people so that tin of tomatoes just went a lot further.

The Nation's Favourite: Spaghetti Bolognaise

Obviously the above is just an example of what I cooked on a particular day and I can't cover every possible example of home cooking without creating a diet book. So, for a further example let's go with something most of us will have eaten or made at some point: Spaghetti Bolognaise. I guarantee that whenever you've eaten 'Spag Bol' in the past you've had a heap of spaghetti with a dollop of bolognaise sauce to accompany it. As spaghetti is dense in carbohydrates it might seem like a challenge to fit this meal into the Fix, Fuel and Fill methodology: Not at all.

Remember, the Final Countdown Diet is not about banning any food so we're not going to come up with a fanciful 'alternative' to spaghetti. Instead we're going to stick to our portion size and fill up the other half of the plate with something else.

That 'something else' is Mediterranean-style vegetables. Prior to starting the rest of the meal I would chop up some courgettes (zucchini), red onions, peppers and aubergines (eggplant) and mix them all together with some dried herbs and olive oil. I would then put the whole lot on a baking tray and shove them in a hot oven so that they can roast through. This is easy to do, doesn't take much time and doesn't require any particular culinary skill. This also forms the Fill Section of the plate and adds some lovely colour to the meal.

Whilst the Mediterranean vegetables are roasting away I can now prepare the sauce and spaghetti to form the Fix and Fuel sections. The protein element will come from lean beef mince or indeed, as an alternative, I might use turkey mince. For the sauce I will use passata or tinned tomatoes instead of sauce from a jar to avoid any unnecessary sugars. I prepare the spaghetti in the normal way and ensure I stick to a tennis ball-sized portion. This completes the Fuel section and is the last element of the meal.

The above ideas are just a suggestion. There are lots of ways you can transform a meal just by adhering to the Fix, Fuel and Fill formula. Why not buy two or three bamboo steamers from a Chinese grocery store (easily available and very cheap) and the next time you're cooking something pile a few different varieties of vegetables into the steamers and let them cook through gently whilst you concentrate on the part of the meal that requires a bit more effort to cook?

Your fridge: Garbage in, Garbage out

No matter what you enjoy cooking and how you decide to stick to the 3F System the main principle is to have your fridge and cupboards filled with all the things you need to stick to the plan. If your fridge is full of fresh produce then that's what you'll end up cooking with. Also, because your plate is going to be full of Fill ingredients, you'll be spending less on expensive cuts of meat. A kilo of vegetables costs a lot less than a kilo of meat. However, if your fridge is full of ready meals then, unfortunately, you may have no choice but to get the fork out and start pricking that cellophane. I guarantee though, following the 3F System will be better for you, will help you lose fat and will also save you money.

PART THREE: MAKING IT HAPPEN

In Part One we discussed some of the hurdles that present themselves when we try to lose weight. We considered the drawbacks of simply counting calories and how exercise can help you lose fat but isn't a solution in itself. We also outlined how, over millions of years of evolution, our body has developed into a supreme fat storage machine. None of these factors are personally unique to you. They apply to everybody. Of course, their impact on you and your efforts to lose fat are uniquely personal.

In Part Two I outlined what I believe to be a very workable eating plan that will lead to long term and sustainable fat loss. Simply put, following the 3F System will result in you losing fat and will help you to keep that fat off. We're not out of the woods yet though. There are a few more things we need to discuss to really make this fat loss happen.

Following hot on the heels of Part Two, this next Part - which I have cunningly called 'Part Three' (see what I did there?) - will provide you with the tips and tools you need to really make a success of the eating plan. It will explore some of the pitfalls that dieters commonly fall into and will give you more appropriate ways of measuring and succeeding in your fat loss goals.

However, no matter how great all of this advice is, it's not worth anything without you. You are the one that's going to make this fat loss happen and you need to be committed to this goal. Importantly, you need to stick at it. I like the quote below from Thomas Edison - the electricity pioneer and inventor of the first practical light bulb.

"Many of life's failures are people who did not realise how close they were to success when they gave up"

To put it another way, if you don't keep on trying you'll never succeed. You're nearly there - on to the last part!

.

DON'T TRUST YOUR SCALES

Here's a scenario you might be familiar with. You start a diet and a few days later you weigh yourself. The weight is dropping off and things are looking good. You can't believe the progress you're making and you feel better in yourself. Your clothes start to feel better. This diet is great and you tell all your friends. You've found a diet that actually works!

A few days later, with the sun shining and a smile on your face you step onto the scales. Your face drops. You can't believe it. You've actually put *on* weight! How can that be? You blame the diet. It's rubbish. You've wasted your time. It's over. Has this ever happened to you? It's happened to me and I can tell you that it wasn't my fault. If the same happened to you it wasn't your fault either. It's the fault of your scales. They are to blame. Don't trust them.

Most scales are dumb

Maybe it's a bit harsh blaming it all on the scales so I'll take a step back from that. Scales might not be untrustworthy – they are however dumb. Why do I think this? When you step on a scale all it does is give you a number. This is obviously your weight. That's all most scales can do. However the aim of any diet is to lose *fat*. In many respects it doesn't matter what you weigh in total. You may well be losing fat but your scales don't know this simply because they are dumb. All they know is one number: your weight.

Your weight isn't as important as you think

The problem is, your body weight isn't just made up of fat. Your body is made up of fat *and* muscle, bones, internal organs, undigested food, lots of internal goo (technical term!) and most relevant of all – water. This combination of things all adds up to your weight. What's more, the balance between all of these components can shift dramatically from day to day and even from hour to hour. Let's have a look at a few scenarios to explain how this can create a problem for you.

Scenario One: You start a diet and start exercising vigorously. You feel better, you're losing weight and you feel healthier. A few days later however you step on the scales and have *gained* weight. Why? One outcome might be that you've been building small amounts of muscle during your exercise regime. Muscle is a dense tissue. A tennis ball sized lump of muscle weighs more than a similar sized blob of fat. It stands to reason therefore that if you're gaining muscle you will need to lose a lot more fat to lose weight.

Scenario Two: It's a few days into your diet and you've experienced some good weight loss. However you find that in the space of 24 hours you've jumped back up in weight. Why? This sort of weight loss may well be due to the water balance within your body. It may be that you've retained some water. There are various reasons for this but, surprisingly, one reason might be that you're not drinking enough. When we drink less our body starts sensing it is in danger of dehydrating. As a survival mechanism it holds on to water until the danger has passed. The solution to this is blindingly obvious. Always drink plenty of water. It doesn't matter if your water comes from a cup of tea as long as you're keeping yourself hydrated.

Scenario Three: You experience a similar sudden weight gain but this time you've been drinking a lot of water lately. The problem here may well be down to salt. If you consume a lot of salt then your body holds on to water. Without going too deep into the science our bodies need a steady concentration of electrolytes to pass messages throughout our body. If we consume salt this increases the electrolyte concentration above normal levels. Our body therefore responds by holding on to water and sending 'I am thirsty' messages to our brain. This is the very reason you find salty snacks in pubs. The more salt you consume, the more drinks you'll buy. The solution is to keep a close eye on your salt intake. Salt lurks in high proportions in processed foods so always check the label. The recommended daily maximum amount is only 6g – about one teaspoon.

Scenario Four: You're on a diet and your weight goes up and down. Nothing in the previous scenarios seems to apply. You've not put on muscle, your water intake is fine and there are no salted peanuts demanding to be eaten. The cause might be your body's glycogen levels. Glycogen acts like a fuel tank releasing energy throughout the day. To store this energy it needs about 1kg of water. During the day this energy gets used and the storage water is released and passes out of you as urine. The good news is that the amount of glycogen in your body is directly linked to how much you weigh. As you lose weight your body will store less glycogen and will therefore hold less water. This benefits you in two ways. Firstly the weight fluctuations will diminish - as the fuel tank gets smaller. Secondly, and even better, when you have a small fuel tank there is less fuel getting stored. This means that once the fuel tank is empty there's only one place left to get more fuel – your body's fat reserves! So losing weight actually helps you to lose weight! Crazy!

So, what does this all mean? It means that you need to feel good about yourself first and foremost and don't worry too much about what the scales say on a daily basis.

When you feel good and you notice small incremental changes – such as your clothes starting to feel more comfortable - this is a sign that your diet is working. You need to look out for and appreciate these signs. But what if you just can't keep away from the scales?

If you must weigh yourself...

One solution, for those of us with a scales addiction, is to buy a set of Body Composition scales. These scales (such as those manufactured by Tanita and other companies) tell you all sorts of information by passing small, unnoticeable, electrical currents through your body as you stand on them. Typically you can measure the percentage of water in your body, your body fat percentage, what your muscles weigh and how much fat is sat around your vital organs. A word of caution however – only use this information as a guide. These aren't medical devices, they're just scales with a few 'bells and whistles' added. They are however useful for determining what has led to any weight shift. For example, if I weigh myself and my weight has increased then I can scroll through the information to find out why. Often it's because the percentage of water in my body has increased. No need to worry unduly – unless of course there are other factors at play such as dehydration.

A good habit to get into is to always weigh yourself at the same time of day. This ensures consistency between readings. A good time to do this is within an hour of waking, after you have had a drink and after you've been to the loo. Obviously what you do on the loo will also make a difference to how much you weigh. This routine ensures you will be hydrated and that any food from the previous evening has more or less disappeared. You should also weigh yourself naked. Try not to do this on a railway platform. Your bathroom is best.

Alternatives to stepping on the scales

OK, so we've decided that scales are not a great way to motivate yourself on a diet because your weight is made up of so many things other than fat. To overcome this you need to become your own human scale. As we've discussed before, a good indicator of fat loss is how your clothes are fitting. If you start to use that extra hole on your belt, or if things just generally feel a bit more comfortable, then you are losing fat. You may also notice changes to your body when looking in the mirror. I say 'may' as it's often too easy to be critical of our bodies and look for the bad things – the lumps and bumps – rather than the good. You need to start looking for the good.

Another factor in determining if a diet is working is how you feel. Do you feel like you have more energy? Do you feel good in yourself? All of these factors are good indicators that you are losing fat and the diet is working. As I mentioned earlier, sometimes it's easy to look in the mirror and tell yourself you're fat. I remember I did this once and walked out of the bathroom feeling like I was a failure. I then put on my jeans and noticed that - for the first time in ages - I had moved up a belt notch. The jeans also felt a lot more comfortable. I was not a failure at all. The diet was working but I had been too critical of myself and was looking for the bad points.

Spending a moment to think about how your clothes are fitting, noticing any signs in the mirror and considering how you feel about yourself will ensure you are focusing on what's actually happening to your body. This paints a far truer picture than those dumb scales.

IN A NUTSHELL

- Scales are dumb. They only know what you weigh. They don't know what that weight is made up of.
- Dehydration, salt and the body's glycogen reserves (the fuel tank) all impact the amount of water your body holds on to. This affects your overall weight.
- If you have to weigh yourself, do it at the same time of day, under the same conditions, after you've been to the loo and do it nude. Avoid public weighing machines when doing this!
- A better indicator of how much fat you are losing can be found in simple things like your clothes fitting better, how you look in the mirror and whether you feel better in yourself.

DON'T TRUST THE BODY MASS
INDEX EITHER

On 17th June 1998 an obesity epidemic, the type of which the world had never seen before, descended on the USA. Millions of Americans woke up on that sunny Wednesday morning to find themselves obese. There had been no warning and there was no way they could avoid it. They simply got out of bed and BAM! They were obese.

A Government-induced obesity epidemic

This epidemic was caused by a US Government Department: The National Institutes of Health. They achieved this by redefining the criteria used to measure a person's Body Mass Index (BMI). Anyone who has ever been weighed by a Doctor will probably know something about the BMI. Generally you are shown a colourful chart that allows you to read your weight against your height. The point at which the weight line intersects the height line will tell you where on the BMI scale you are. Your point on the scale then identifies you as underweight, normal, overweight or obese.

From 'normal' to 'overweight' in 24 hours

What the National Institutes of Health did on that Wednesday in June 1998 was to lower the starting weight for all categories. In some instances the starting weight was lowered by as much as 10lbs (approx. 4.5kg). The result of lowering the weights meant that more people became overweight or obese.

Take for example a person previously considered within the 'normal' range. From that Wednesday onwards they might need to drop another 4.5kg to remain in that category. This change to the BMI's criteria led to 29 million American citizens being re-defined as overweight. What's more, a year or so later the World Health Organisation did exactly the same thing and made millions of people around the world overweight!

Some people just happen to be heavy

In addition to the idiocy of what happened above, there are other problems with the BMI. Let me tell you something about me: I've always been heavy. In the last chapter we discussed how weight doesn't always equate to being fat. In my circumstance this is generally true. I'm just one of those heavy guys who weighs more than he should do. Several years ago my wife and I had our first child - a boy called William. This little chap shares a lot of my own bodily characteristics. He has the same long body and short legs (I appreciate this doesn't paint a wonderful mental picture). In all respects he's a 'Mini Me'. When William was about 2 years old I noticed something very interesting that set him apart from children of a similar age.

I noticed that other parents found William to be mind-blowingly heavy.

We've all been to parties and seen parents lifting kids on to climbing frames etc. When it came to William's turn the same scenario played out time-after-time. The Dad would grab hold of William, start the lift and typically stop in mid air. The Dad would then normally utter an expletive under his breath and comment about how heavy William was. The stronger Dads would carry on and lift him however some would just give up (this *happened!*). You see William *is* heavy. He's not overweight – he's a healthy and active child. However he takes after me and I'm heavy. But guess what, the BMI says I'm overweight and it will say the same for William when he gets older. Can you imagine how constantly being told you're overweight might affect someone who is in a healthy weight range? It won't help them - that's for sure.

Who wants to settle for average?

The main fault with the BMI is that it works on averages. Averages are great if you're conducting some big population study and want to see how the inhabitants of one whole town compare with those of another. Averages however are not very good for use at an individual level. The BMI therefore has problems dealing with people who are tall, people who are lean and people who are athletic and have high muscle mass. In 2008 a study concluded that the accuracy of the BMI in diagnosing obesity was limited[35]. The study published in the International Journal of Obesity found that not only did the BMI misclassify people with normal levels of fat as overweight; it also classified a high proportion of people with excess body fat as being normal. The wider implication of this is that health resources might get directed in the wrong direction.

So what use is the BMI?

If it's so inaccurate, then why is the BMI used at all? The answer is simple. Basically it is easy to use, easy to understand and nobody has come up with a better alternative. This argument is a bit like saying that if spoons didn't exist a fork would be the ideal way to eat soup. Using something that isn't fit for purpose doesn't make it right! Admittedly, the BMI does have some use. It is at its best when dealing with extremes of body weight: the chronically overweight or the chronically underweight. My guess is that a Doctor would be able to tell if a patient fell into any of those categories the moment they walked through the door!

So, what does this mean to you? Unless you fit into one of the two extremes of body weight then I don't think you should get hung up on your BMI level. I've been overweight all my life according to the BMI and, although it was certainly correct for a number of years, it's been wrong a lot more often than it's been right. Never at any time in my life has my BMI score affected how good or how bad I feel about myself. I didn't let it. The way we feel about ourselves and how our clothes fit is a more accurate indicator of fat loss. Don't let the BMI put a downer on all the hard work you're putting into your body.

IN A NUTSHELL

- The BMI can classify people as obese who aren't obese. Some people are naturally heavier than others but the BMI can't spot this.

- The BMI is useful if you want to identify if you're extremely obese or extremely skinny. But you'll probably know if you're in one of those categories anyway.

- Don't use the BMI to track any progress you've made losing fat because the BMI only works on weight. We know weight is made up of lots of other things in addition to fat.

- If your clothes fit better, you're looking good in the mirror and you feel happier – who cares what the BMI says anyway!

GETTING YOUR BRAIN INTO GEAR

My wife Jane was staring at her wardrobe complaining that she was cramming too many clothes into too small a space. 'They're all getting crumpled' she grumbled. It had been two years since our daughter had been born and six months since Jane had shed the post-baby fat she had put on. In that time she had gone down a dress size or two (depending on which shop she bought the clothes from!).

'Why are you keeping all the bigger clothes?' I asked 'are you planning to put the fat back on again?' Jane thought for a moment and decided not to hurl a coat hanger at me. She realised I was just trying to be helpful - in a clumsy and unintentionally insulting sort of way. 'Good point' she said, and with that started the process of bundling her outsize clothes off to the charity shop.

Now, this was an important act in more ways than one. First, the physical act of getting rid of the larger clothes sent an important message to Jane's brain. She was telling herself there was no way she was ever going back to wearing those bigger clothes again. Perhaps more importantly, she had no option of switching back to the larger clothes if she grew bigger in the future.

Wear clothes that are the 'right' size

Jane also now had a good physical measure of the size she needed to stay at. All her clothes were now the right size. Every time she got dressed in the morning she would unconsciously gauge how comfortable her clothes were. If they felt a bit tight the only way to rectify this would be to amend her diet to lose a bit of fat. Maybe this would start with a smaller breakfast and continue throughout the day. I have had similar experiences when my jeans needed loosening by an extra belt notch to fit comfortably.

Rectify small gains in fat by small changes to your routine

You may well be incredulous at the above and might think it's all a bit simplistic. However all we're doing is keeping an eye out for the first signs of our body fat starting to move in the wrong direction. The alternative is to invest in a tape measure and a set of body fat calipers so you can take daily readings. I much prefer the simple route. Why complicate things?

The overall aim of this is to nip any change in the bud early on so it's easier to rectify. This doesn't mean you have to take any drastic action. Small and incremental changes to your daily routine are enough to have an effect. Maybe you need to consider how well you've stuck to the 3F System recently? Perhaps you need to take the stairs instead of the lift? Whatever you choose to do you don't have to resort to willpower, hypnotism or anything else. You just need to notice what's happening to your body and start tweaking things to help you to lose fat.

Realise any willpower you have will soon be gone

On the subject of willpower, the first thing you need to be aware of is that willpower is of extremely limited use when you want to lose fat. In fact, willpower isn't going to help you much at all. The problem with willpower is that it can only last as long as you can focus on the outcome. As soon as that focus drops you have lost the willpower.

In much the same way as your body becomes fatigued by strenuous exercise, willpower weakens the more often it is used. A number of scientific studies have shown that people who have successfully used willpower on one occasion have a real problem using it for a second time[36]. Put another way, if you are on a diet that 'forbids' certain foods your willpower will inevitably weaken and you'll end up raiding the metaphorical cookie jar. The result is that the diet has failed. Note: it is the *diet* that has failed and not *you*. The fact is, willpower was never going to work.

Here's another story from my experience. A friend of mine, let's call her Karen, wanted to lose fat for a holiday. Karen really wanted the bikini body we've spoken about before. She chose what people often think is the easy route. She enrolled on one of those diets where the 'meals' are sachets of powder mixed with water. Karen wanted to lose fat so badly that when she was invited to a wedding she took along her sachets and ate those instead of the food put on by the bride and groom (poached salmon and green veg – a nice healthy meal). The result of this willpower, in sticking to the sachets, was that Karen did indeed lose some weight (I use the term 'weight' and not 'fat' on purpose) and went on holiday feeling better about herself. However the story doesn't end there.

Karen's chosen holiday was at an all-inclusive resort. "Oh no!" I hear you gasp. Guess what? Faced with an abundance of tempting food, Karen put all her weight back on. You could argue that her aim was to just lose weight for the holiday and that was OK. However I know Karen and the sad fact is, that wasn't her aim. Her aim was to lose fat and to lose fat permanently. She thought the sachets would be the quick fix she needed for a slimmer body. They weren't. In fact all they did was put her back to square one. Karen is only now beginning to lose fat by following the Final Countdown Diet. Quick fix diets do not work.

Focus on the outcome, not the timeframe

The above is a salutary lesson; it is vital that you start

your diet by forgetting about the 'Quick Fix'. Losing fat is a long-term process. Following the Final Countdown Diet will result in some immediate benefits however fat loss has to take place consistently over a long period of time for it to be permanent. Remember, your body has a set baseline weight it thinks you should weigh. You can only change your body's thinking gradually. Tiny footsteps will allow your body to lower the baseline. Sprinting in and expecting immediate results won't work. You simply can't rush it.

Think about some of the questions I posed at the start of the book – in particular about celebrity diets. Some magazines seem to survive on stories about famous people getting thin. But what happens once the paid-for nutritionists and personal trainers have left the celebrity's home? You'll find out if you pick up the same magazine a few months later. In all likelihood you'll see an unflattering photo of the celebrity on a beach and a headline gasping about how much weight she's gained. This will be followed by another diet in a month or two with the magazine keeping you informed of her progress. This is classic yo-yo dieting. Just think, if a celebrity with untold resources at their disposal can't keep the weight off then something must be wrong with the process. That 'something' is the mind-set that you can lose fat both quickly *and* permanently.

The choice is yours but only one answer makes sense

Here is the truth. You can either opt for short-term fat loss *or* permanent fat loss. However you can only have one

– you can't have both. You need to get yourself comfortable with this fact. Do you want to lose fat just for a short while or do you want to lose fat permanently? The problem with today's consumer society is that we want and expect everything to be immediately available. Our bodies however live in the Stone Age and haven't cottoned on to this. Sure, rapid fat loss sounds appealing – but what about the following month when it's all come back on again? Permanent fat loss is by far the better alternative. To achieve this you should avoid giving yourself an unrealistic timeframe and should instead take comfort in the signs that you are gradually improving. I guarantee with such focus you will be in a better place in 6 months time than you would be if you jumped onto every 'quick fix' diet currently available.

'Starvation' dieting leads to binge eating

You may have noticed throughout the book that I attach a lot of importance to flexibility, choice and not being too restrictive in following the Final Countdown Diet. There are very good reasons for this. Research has shown that people who are constantly dieting tend to overeat when they are faced with a large choice of food[37]. This is because restrictive diets rely on willpower to keep you away from forbidden foods. As we discussed earlier, willpower doesn't last forever.

The Final Countdown Diet has been formulated to remove total reliance on willpower. Of course, there are some 'rules' but they're not designed to be absolute. There's enough 'breathing space' in there so you don't feel like you're being punished for wanting to lose fat. The occasional sugary treat or processed food is fine - as long as it's truly occasional it's not going to create a major problem. You should however take some steps to avoid being tempted back to making these foods a mainstay of your diet. How can you avoid this?

Give your cupboards a spring clean

The first thing we need to do is change our environment. No, I don't mean we need to install windmills in our gardens or put solar panels on our roof. What I mean is we need to remove from our reach those things that are just so impossibly tempting that whenever we see them we have to eat them – and continue eating them until they're all gone. You know the culprits: biscuits, chocolates, whatever it might be. If you've just read this and are thinking 'I'll do that as soon as I've finished that packet of cookies in the cupboard' then give yourself a mental slap around the face! Do it now (getting rid of the cookies, not the slap!). Which would you rather lose – fat or a few biscuits?

The next thing we can do is stock our shelves and cupboards with all the good things we're going to be eating whilst following the 3F System: vegetables and pulses and suchlike. This way, when we go to the cupboard to decide on what to cook we only find good things in there.

If you're a shopper who gets seduced by all the offers in the supermarket and grabs anything that's Buy-One-

Get-One-Free then maybe it's time you started to shop online and have your groceries delivered to your home. This way you can avoid the temptation of stocking up on copious amounts of food that will either get eaten or wasted. I find that I can save money on my weekly shop by doing this – even when the delivery cost is taken into account. It also means I can spend the time at home that I would've spent pushing a trolley around the aisles.

Closely linked to the above paragraph is planning. If you plan ahead for what you are going to eat in the week then there is less chance of you having to 'make do' with any unhealthy choices lurking in your cupboards. This is especially important if you've ignored previous advice and kept your cupboards stocked with unhealthy things. You need to take control of what you eat – don't let your cupboards dictate to you!

Eating healthily is a habit you will learn to love

Can you train your brain to prefer healthy foods above unhealthy foods? Yes you absolutely can! A study in America found that when obese adults were put on a food education and healthy diet programme something happened to their brains[38]. Over a 6-month period their brains began to become more sensitive to the reward and enjoyment to be derived from healthier food. In conjunction, their brains became less sensitive to reward from unhealthy food. Put simply, the guys being studied started to really enjoy healthy food and found unhealthy food to be less tempting. Over a relatively short period of time they'd begun to think, act and eat more healthily without any real conscious effort other than being educated to good food choices and following a diet plan. This is basically what I have tried to achieve with the Final Countdown Diet.

Nobody is perfect

As I mentioned briefly before, The Final Countdown Diet has been formulated to give you enough breathing space so you don't have to rely totally on willpower. Nobody can be 'perfect'100% of the time. It would be a very boring world if we were. At times you will fall off the plan and tuck into something unhealthy. I guarantee it. However this really doesn't matter as long as you aim to eat healthily and follow the Plan's guidelines for 80-90% of the time. Why beat yourself up and feel guilty about that slice of cake? Enjoy the moment and get back onto track the next opportunity you have. You don't have to write off the whole day for one extravagant lunch. You can make amends at the very next meal. As long as falling off the plan doesn't become a daily habit then you'll be absolutely fine. Life is for living so go out there and live it!

IN A NUTSHELL

- As you lose fat – lose your old clothes. Your new clothes will become a surrogate set of scales and an easy to use tape measure to help keep an eye on your fat loss progress.

- Correcting small short-term gains in fat is easier to do

in the short-term. Long-term gains take a lot longer.

- Your focus should be on the end result – permanent fat loss. Don't burden yourself with unrealistic expectations of short-term rapid fat loss.

- Willpower is not going to work – no matter how well intentioned you start out.

- Change your food environment at home to get rid of any indulgent foods that you know won't do you any good.

- In line with the above point, stock up your shelves with healthy 3F System foods and plan out your weekly meals.

- There will be times when you sneak in an indulgent treat. That's life! Live with it and make amends at the next meal.

THE FAQ SUMMARY BIT

This is the 'In a Nutshell' to end all Nutshells! The following few pages contain many of the principles of the Final Countdown Diet Plan in FAQ format for easy reference. The aim of this is to be a memory jogger – it's not meant to get you out of reading the rest of the book (so go back and read the rest if you haven't already!).

As I mentioned at the start of the book, losing fat is about much more than what you choose to eat. Permanent fat loss not only involves excellent nutrition, it also needs you to be physically and mentally prepared for the fat loss journey. This is why a lot of diets fail. They focus solely on the food and ignore the daily life you lead. For some reason they ignore the fact that you might not want to spend the rest of your life eating Cabbage Soup (for e.g.). Once you 'fail' to meet their diet's unrealistic expectations you feel a failure. You're not a failure; their diet has failed *you*.

I want you to put any images of failure out of your mind. You are about to start on a marvellous journey that will lead to you losing fat and keeping that fat off. It will take time – but you're prepared for that and aren't expecting immediate results. You will however start to feel the benefits almost immediately and you will build on these early benefits as you progress along the road to your ideal body.

Over time you will start to feel more comfortable and will begin having more energy. Quite simply you'll feel a lot better about yourself. There will however be times when you have a 'blow out' and fall off the Plan – sometimes spectacularly. However you realise that this is only natural and it's no big deal. On those occasions you'll simply carry on with the Plan at the next available opportunity. Life is meant to be fun and you wouldn't be human if you didn't allow yourself a guilty pleasure every now and then. With that in mind, let's finish with a few questions and answers about all the things we've discussed in this book.

WHAT'S THE AIM OF ALL THIS?

You need to keep in mind throughout your fat loss journey that your single, solitary and most important aim is PERMANENT FAT LOSS. It's in capitals because it just didn't seem important enough in lower case. What does this mean? It means that you want to lose fat and you want to keep that fat off – forever.

This is important firstly because if you want a quick-fix to lose 'weight' (note: I said 'weight' not 'fat') rapidly that will only result in you putting it all back on again just as quickly – then the Final Countdown Plan is not for you. It's also important because you need to get your head around the idea that sometimes the things you desire take time. You didn't gain fat overnight and you're not going to lose it overnight either. Start off your fat loss process with an understanding that permanent fat loss will take time. However it will be more satisfying and achievable than a hundred quick-fix diets. A journey of a thousand miles starts with a single footstep. You can make that first step today.

WHAT ABOUT DOING A QUICK-FIX DIET BEFORE I START?

Although I can see the rationale for this – you lose weight rapidly and then try to keep it off whilst losing a bit more – unfortunately this won't work. It won't work for all the evolutionary reasons outlined in this book. Once you embark on a quick-fix rapid diet your body is looking out for any sign that you've 'found' food again (remember, your body will think you're suffering in a time of famine). Once you start to eat normally your body will do all it can to get back to its baseline weight. Even if you're eating healthily, you will still put on weight! I can't say this often enough - you didn't gain weight overnight and it's not going to be lost overnight either. The fat loss journey however can start right now with the Final Countdown Diet.

WHEN SHOULD I START?

Start when it's right for you. You don't live in a bubble and at certain times of year the diet industry will bombard you with adverts to tempt you to buy their products. If these times of the year aren't right for you, then don't start your diet. You're not a machine and there may be very good personal reasons why the time isn't right. You should only begin the Final Countdown Diet Plan when you are ready to make the commitment to achieving permanent fat loss.

This is important because you need to embrace the Plan wholly in the initial stages. Psychologists say that it takes 21 days for us to form a habit. You need to make the Final Countdown Diet Plan and the 3F System your new habit. Once you've learnt the basics and followed the Plan for a few weeks then it will become second nature. There's nothing particularly onerous or restrictive about the Final Countdown Diet. It's just good nutritional sense, healthy eating and moderate activity – with the right frame of mind.

SHOULD I BE COUNTING CALORIES?

The first thing to bear in mind is that not all calories are the same. The foods you eat interact with your body in different ways. Calories from sugars will end up getting stored as fat. Calories from vegetables will come loaded with other nutrients that will help your body to flourish. Blindly counting calories is not going to help you.

Calories can however be useful in some situations, such as when determining the right portion size for a breakfast cereal. Many cereals have nutritional information and serving sizes that are appropriate only for children. If you fill your normal-sized breakfast bowl with such a cereal then you will probably be consuming more calories than you realise. In such a situation you need to aim for a calorific target and weigh out an appropriate amount of cereal to meet that target. Using the same bowl each day will help you to decide the optimum fill level.

As a general rule however, you don't need to count calories, just follow the food guidelines within the Fix, Fuel & Fill System and you'll be eating a nutritionally balanced diet that will help you to lose fat.

WHAT DO I NEED TO KNOW ABOUT NUTRITION?

Let's face it, nutrition can be a pretty boring subject. There's a lot of science involved and it's much more fun eating something that it is to read about it. What follows therefore is a very basic summary of what you need to know:

- Proteins fix our body when it is damaged

and they help us to grow. Proteins can be found in varying degrees in eggs, beef, chicken, tuna, lentils and oats

- Carbohydrates are basically sugars. Lots of foods contain carbohydrates and you need a good level of them to give your body the fuel it needs to go about it's daily routine. Too many carbs and your body will probably want to store them as fat. To avoid this you need to eat fewer carbs from starchy foods such as potatoes, rice and beans.

- Fats have had a lot of bad press. Don't worry about these at all. There is a difference between the fat you eat and the fat around your waist.

- Fibre is a good thing to include in your diet. It helps your body efficiently use the carbs you've eaten whilst also filling you up so you don't have to eat as much.

- Vitamins and Minerals don't have to come in pill form. You can get all you need from a balanced diet.

WHY DO I NORMALLY FIND IT DIFFICULT TO LOSE FAT?

The short answer is because you're a human being. Humans are genetically built to hold on to fat. This is a survival mechanism for times of famine.

Your brain also employs several tricks to hold your weight at a level it thinks will protect you from starving. If you start to drastically cut the amount of food you consume then your brain kicks in to hold onto your fat reserves. If you go on a crash diet and then start eating 'normally' your body will use all its resources to get you back to the level it thinks you should weigh. To get around these problems you need to employ a longer-term strategy to lose fat. Quick-fix diets don't work.

I'M GOING TO HIT THE GYM UNTIL I BURN MY FAT OFF. GOOD OR BAD?

Exercise is good for you but it's not the best way of losing fat. If you expend too much energy in the gym your body will want you to replace that with food. You will literally 'work up an appetite'.

If you haven't exercised in a while then a programme of moderate exercise is probably going to give you more benefit than diving straight on to the rowing machine. Small and simple changes to your daily activity levels will make a positive impact on the amount of fat you lose. A walk to the shops or taking the stairs instead of the escalator will all reap rewards. When considering exercise, think small before you think big.

WHAT'S THE FIX, FUEL & FILL SYSTEM?

To avoid calorie counting and to ensure you eat a balanced diet you should imagine your plate is divided into three sections. The first quarter is called 'Fix' and contains Proteins such as meat or poultry. The second quarter is called 'Fuel' and consists of dense carbohydrates such as those found in starchy foods like potatoes or rice. The remaining half of the plate is the 'Fill' section and consists of all other vegetables that have lower carb levels. Refer back to the *Introducing The 3F System* Chapter for a comprehensive breakdown of the type of foods to be found in each section.

It is important when following the 3F System to allow yourself 20 minutes after a meal before considering any second helpings. This gives your brain time to realise you've eaten. If you're still hungry any second helpings need to come solely from the 'Fill' Section.

DO I HAVE ANY ALTERNATIVES?

The 3F System is built around the three main meals of the day and can be applied to each equally. There will be times however when you are rushing about and it may not be convenient to apply a methodical approach to your meal. For many people the busiest times of the day are likely to be at breakfast and lunch times. I have therefore suggested quick and easy options for these meals that fit within the 3F Framework.

BREAKFAST: There are two main options, one is eggs on toast with the toast prepared as discussed in the *Breakfast and Lunch* Chapter. The second option is a bowl of Oats preferably prepared with hot water. The rationale for these choices and much more information can be found in the relevant chapter.

LUNCH: There's one clear lunch-time winner that will help fill you up and lose fat. That winner is Soup. Again, lots more information and the rationale can be found in the *Breakfast and Lunch* Chapter.

WHEN SHOULD I EAT?

The simple answer is that you should eat when you feel the *need* to eat. This might seem obvious but it's not. Throughout the day you will feel the 'desire' to eat and the 'need' to eat. These things are very different. The desire to eat can be sparked by seeing a nice looking cake in a shop window or by the smell of food on a grill. The need to eat however is caused by your body telling you you're actually hungry and you should do something about it.

You have to start recognising these signs. Wherever possible you should move away from set meal times and only eat when your body tells you it's time. This isn't about starvation or unrealistically extending the periods between meals, it's simply about being aware that we often eat when we don't actually need to. Over a period of time the result of this unnecessary eating will inevitably be a few extra inches on your waistline.

CAN I HAVE A SNACK?

Snacks are perfectly acceptable if you find yourself with

a hunger pang that just won't go away. It happens. Your best snack options will be high in protein. Such snacks will ensure you will feel fuller for longer. Good options are nuts such as Almonds, hazelnuts or peanuts. High protein Yoghurt has also been found to keep you fuller for longer and can also prevent you eating loads at your next meal.

WHAT ARE THE BEST DRINKS FOR LOSING FAT?

Refer to the *Drinks and Snacks* Chapter for all the back up information but, in summary, the best drinks for losing fat are: Green Tea, Black Tea or Coffee – all to be taken without milk.

ARE ANY FOODS 'BANNED'?

The Final Countdown Diet is not about banning foods. It's about making better food choices. Can you stick to the diet by regularly eating sugary snacks and highly processed foods? No. Can the occasional sugary snack or highly processed food form part of your diet? Absolutely!

The problem with banning foods is that they instantly become more desirable. For some reason we always want what we can't have!

Some foods you do however need to watch out for, these are foods that typically have a very high carbohydrate content. The most common foods are those containing flour (such as bread, cakes etc) and pastas. Again, these foods aren't banned you just need to be mindful of them and ensure you don't make them an everyday part of your diet.

HOW OFTEN SHOULD I WEIGH MYSELF?

Rarely! The aim here is to lose fat. The problem is your body is made up of many things that constitute your weight. Your overall weight is not just made up of fat – it includes water, muscle, bone etc. Retaining a bit of water doesn't mean your diet isn't working!

If you can't live without weighing yourself then try to get hold of a set of Body Composition Scales and record the various readings. This will give you an indicator of where your weight is heading and will tell you what's causing any weight shift.

A far better indicator of how well your diet is going is the way your clothes fit and how well you feel about yourself.

ANY OTHER BITS OF ADVICE?

As we briefly discussed above, weighing yourself can sometimes be counter-productive. Why not let your clothes tell you how your diet is going? If your clothes are starting to fit better then it's a sure sign you're losing fat. Conversely if your clothes are starting to get tighter then you need to make some adjustments to your daily routine to get back on track with your fat loss.

Another thing you need to be aware of is that willpower and self-control will not work in the long-term. This is why the Final Countdown Diet is pretty relaxed about the odd transgression. You *will* fall off the diet every now and then and have a blow out. This is natural, it's human nature and it is to be celebrated and enjoyed. All you have to do is jump back on the Plan at the next eating occasion. Just as one swallow doesn't make a summer, swallowing a sponge cake doesn't break a diet!

There are lots of great foods that you can eat whilst following the 3F System. Food doesn't have to be boring to be healthy. The chances are you're already eating these foods already but haven't had a system to follow that puts them in their proper place on the plate. To get your diet off to a great start why not stock up your fridge and cupboards with all the great things you're going to eat on the Final Countdown Diet Plan? Eating should be fun after all!

EPILOGUE

I love the word 'epilogue'. It used to crop up at the end of rubbish American Detective shows when I was little. I never knew what it meant but figured out it was like a conclusion to the show. Just when you thought the show was over the magical word 'Epilogue' would appear. You'd then find out what happened to all the characters after the show's story had been told. It was the Director's way of saying 'I've wasted enough of your time and I really can't think of another way of telling you all this quickly so here's a few bullet points'. It served its purpose. We were glad the bad guy had been punished and the victim was now happy. What follows is my epilogue.

We've been through a lot of information in this book. I've tried to tell you everything I know about the diet industry and how to eat healthily in a format I hope you found interesting and enjoyable. I've also told you a bit about myself. I told you at the outset that during the few years I spent in China I put on a lot of fat. This gain in fat necessarily sparked my interest in the world of dieting. It occurred to me in writing this book that China was, in fact, a long time ago. I decided there was only one way I could categorically prove that the fat loss system I had developed still worked. So I went back to China and went back to my old decadent ways.

Shortly after completing the manuscript for this book I booked a flight to China. My objectives were twofold. The first objective was to catch up with old friends. The second objective was to eat like a little piggy! Soon after I arrived I had my first food blowout. I was at a restaurant and basically ordered three main courses just for me. I continued with similar blowouts for an intensive 3-week period. I knew this wasn't going to do me much good – but that was the point. I even went to a restaurant where if you ate their 3kg (yes, 3kg!) burger you didn't have to pay. In hindsight I'm glad I failed.

Throughout this period I intentionally threw all the FCD principles out of the window. This was my experiment to see how rock solid those principles are. Without exception every meal consisted of a minimum of three dishes washed down with a few bottles of beer. I ate until I was full and then waited a couple of hours before starting all over again. It wasn't big or clever but I knew that it was something I had to do.

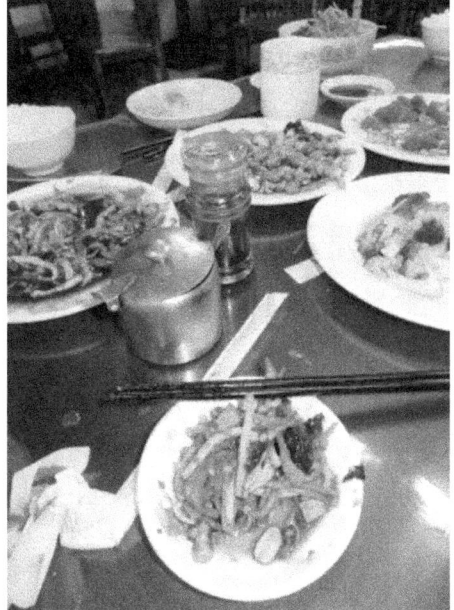

Snacking: Beijing Style

When I returned home I weighed myself. In just three weeks I had put on almost 2kg of weight! Using my body composition scales I could see that most of this was either body fat or visceral fat – the fat surrounding the body's organs. Not good. In hindsight the whole idea was a bit hazardous to health and insanely foolish.

Once I was settled back home I immediately stepped back onto the FCD Plan. I didn't find reverting back to my FCD habits difficult in the slightest. These habits were more ingrained in me than a few weeks of madness. The weight slowly began to drop off and this continued even though my return coincided with a hectic period of birthday parties and visiting friends. That's the beauty of the FCD Plan. You can take part in such events as long as you stick to the principles when filling your buffet plate. You won't look or feel out of place and you'll keep on losing weight.

Just under four weeks after returning from China I had lost all that extra weight and my body and visceral fat percentages were back to their previous levels. The rate of weight loss - approximately 500g/week – is widely acknowledged as being safe and sustainable. A few months later and I'm still at my comfortable weight and I'm happy that my clothes are fitting me better than they did previously.

So, this is my epilogue. It's what happened to me after I finished the book. I went back to where it all started and did the Final Countdown Diet all over again. I appreciate that you may be looking at a challenge of losing more than 'just' 2kg of fat but whatever fat you have to lose – you need to realise that it *is* achievable. You just need to be honest with yourself. Putting on fat didn't happen overnight and getting rid of it also isn't going to happen overnight. Follow the guidelines in this book and I assure you that as of tomorrow you will be one day closer to being your dream size.

Now it's time for you to create your own epilogue. I'd really love to know what happened to you after you finished the book. This book has a website, www.finalcountdowndiet.com which I hope can be a forum for us to share ideas, experiences and support each other. I hope you will visit the site to share your experiences and I wish you every success in following the Final Countdown Diet. Take Care, God Bless and Live Happy. Life's too short to be counting calories!

Will Meadows
West Yorkshire
Autumn 2014

ABOUT WILL MEADOWS

Will Meadows was born and grew up in a once-proud South Yorkshire town. Much of his working life has been spent travelling the globe and he has a particular fondness for Asia.

His career has spanned a number of industries with the majority of his experience in the fields of diet and nutrition.

Will has authored a number of magazine and journal articles. A distillation of Will's personal and working experiences can be found in The Final Countdown Diet.

Will lives in West Yorkshire in a village closely linked with food. He lives with his wife Jane and their three children. Will speaks, and eats, Chinese.

STILL NEED CONVINCING THIS WORKS?

I've tried to gather together as much information as I can to back up or illustrate the points I make in this book. I think it's important that you know that my comments are not just the rants of a deranged madman!

Where possible I have sought out the most recent research. The majority of the papers referred to can easily be found online by searching the author or the title. Some papers are however from specialist journals that can only be accessed by subscription. It's worth seeing if your local library can access these for you if they are of particular interest.

Many popular diets don't result in long-term weight loss

[1] Eisenberg M, Atallah R et al (2014) "Long-term benefits of popular diets are less than evident" *Circulation: Cardiovascular Quality and Outcomes* Nov 14

Some proteins are better than others

[2] Protein Quality Evaluation: Report of Joint FAO/WHO Expert Consultation. Food and Nutrition Paper 51. Rome, 1991.

Eating foods with a low carb density is better than just following a low carb diet

[3] Spreadbury, Ian (2012) "Comparison with ancestral diets suggests dense acellular carbohydrates promote an inflammatory microbiota, and may be the primary dietary cause of leptin resistance and obesity" *Diabetes, Metabolic Syndrome and Obesity: Targets and Therapy 4 July 2012*

Reducing fat doesn't reduce your waistline

[4] Heini, Adrian & Weinsier, Roland (1997) "Divergent trends in obesity and fat intake patters: The american paradox": *The American Journal of Medicine vol 102 p 259-264 March 1997*

Eating Fat doesn't make you fat

[5] Ebbeling C.B., Leidig M.M., Feldman H.A., Lovesky M.M., and D.S. Ludwig. (2007). Effects of a low-glycemic load vs low-fat diet in obese young adults: A randomized trial. *Journal of the American Medical Association.* 297(19):2092-102

Most people who diet will regain the weight they have lost

[6] Sumithran, P & Proietto, J (2013) "The defence of body weight: a physiological basis for weight regain after weight loss": *Clinical Science (2013) 124*

Your body has a set baseline for what it thinks is your ideal weight

[7] Muller, M, Bosy-Westphal, A & Heymsfield, S (2010) "Is there evidence for a set point that regulates human body weight?": *F1000 Med Rep; 2:59*

If you lose fat this results in low levels of leptin which leads to your brain telling you to eat more

[8] Muller, M, Bosy-Westphal, A & Heymsfield, S (2010) "Is there evidence for a set point that regulates human body weight?": *F1000 Med Rep; 2:59*

Losing weight on a diet makes you hungrier and makes you crave high calorie foods
[9] Sumithran, P & Proietto, J (2013) "The defence of body weight: a physiological basis for weight regain after weight loss": *Clinical Science (2013) 124*

Who says that walking is a good form of exercise?

[10] Wilkin, LD, Cheryl, A & Haddock BL (2012) "Energy expenditure comparison between walking and running in average fitness individuals": *The Journal of Strength and Conditioning Research 2012 Apr 26(4)*

If you consume fructose then moderate exercise will offset the health risks

[11] Bidwell, AJ, Fairchild TJ, Redmond J et al (2014) "Physical activity offsets the negative effects of a high-fructose diet": *Medicine and Science in Sports Exercise 2014 Nov;46(11)*

Surely intense aerobic exercise is better than a walk to the shops?

[12] Andersen R, Wadden T, Bartlett S, Zemel B, Verde T & Franckowiak SC (1999) "Effect of lifestyle activity vs structured aerobic exercise in obese women: a randomized trial": *The Journal of the American Medical Association 1999 Jan 27;281(4)*

What do you mean, fidgeting can help me lose weight?

[13] Levine, J, Schleusner S & Jensen M (2000) "Energy Expenditure of nonexercise activity": *The American Journal of Clinical Nutrition Dec 2000 72*

Eating a lot of smaller meals doesn't make you lose weight

[14] Cameron JD, Cyr MJ and Doucet E (2010) "Increased meal frequency does not promote greater weight loss in subjects who were prescribed an 8-week equi-energetic energy-restricted diet." *British Journal of Nutrition, 2010 Apr; 103(8): 1098-101*

Eating a lot of smaller meals might actually make you feel hungrier

[15] Ohkawara K, Cornier MA, Kohrt WM & Melanson EL (2013) "Effects of increased meal frequency on fat oxidation and perceived hunger". *Obesity (Silver Spring) 2013 Feb: 21(2) 336-43*

Black Tea helps to reduce or prevent obesity

[16] Satoshi U, Yoshimasa T & Akiko Saka et al (2010) "Prevention of diet-induced obesity by dietary black tea

polyphenols extract in vitro and in vivo" *Nutrition.* Vol 27, Issue 3: 287-292

Milky tea stops you from losing fat

[17] Research conducted by Devajit Borthakur, a scientist at the Tea Research Association in Assam, India in 2011 (various online sources)

Green Tea helps you burn off more energy

[18] Westerterp-Plantenga MS (2010) "Green tea catechins, caffeine and body-weight regulation" *Physiology & Behaviour.* 2010 Apr 26:100(1):42-6

When you lose weight, green tea helps you to keep it off

[19] Hursel R, Viechtbauer W, Westerterp-Plantega MS (2009) "The effects of green tea on weight loss and weight maintenance: a meta-analysis". *International Journal of Obesity (London)* 2009 Sep:33(9):956-61

Caffeine makes you alert, gives you energy and helps you to concentrate

[20] Chawla J, Lorenzo N & Suleman A et al (2013) "Neurologic Effects of Caffeine." *Medscape Aug 12, 2013.*

Diet drinks might make you gain fat

[21] Swithers S (2013) "Artificial Sweeteners Produce the Counter-Intuitive Effect of Inducing Metabolic Derangements." *Trends in Endocrinology & Metabolism* Vol 24, Issue 9, Sep 2013: 431-441

Eating yoghurt as a snack will fill you up and stop you eating loads in your next meal

[22] Ortinau L, Hoertel H, Douglas S & Leidy H (2014) *"Effects of high-protein vs. high-fat snacks on appetite control, satiety, and eating initiation in healthy women"* Nutrition Journal 2014, 13:97

Chocolate is a fat-busting miracle food (in very small quantities) ...probably

[23] Farhat G, Drummond S, Fyfe L & Al-Dujaili EA (2014) *"Dark Chocolate: an obesity paradox or a culprit for weight gain?"* Phytotherapy Research 2014 Jun: 28(6):791-7

Freezing your bread before it's toasted lowers the GI of the bread

[24] Burton P & Lightowler HJ (2008) "The impact of freezing and toasting on the glycaemic response of white bread". *European Journal of Clinical Nutrition* 62, 594-599

Eggs keep you fuller for longer

[25] Vander Wal JS, Marth JM, Khosla P, Jen K-LC & Dhurandhar NV (2005) "Short term effect of eggs on satiety in overweight and obese subjects". *Journal of the American College of Nutrition* 245: 510-515

Eating an egg breakfast helps with weight loss

[26] Vander Wal JS, Gupta A, Khosla P, Dhurandhar NV (2008) "Egg breakfast enhances weight loss". *International Journal of Obesity* 32: 1545 - 1551

Oats are great to have at breakfast: they control your appetite and keep you full

[27] Rebello CJ, Johnson WD & Martin CK et al (2013) "Acute effect of oatmeal on subjective measures of appetite and satiety compared to a ready-to-eat breakfast cereal: a randomized crossover trial." *Journal of the American College of Nutrition* 2013:32(4):272-9

If you eat Oats you will eat less at your next meal because you're full

[28] Beck E, Tosh SM, Batterham MJ, Tapsell LC & Huang XF (2009) "Oat beta-glucan increases postprandial cholecystokinin levels, decreases insulin response and extends subjective satiety in overweight subjects." *Molecular Nutrition & Food Research.* 2009 Oct; 53(10):1343-51

Soup eaters are thinner

[29] Zhu Y & Hollis JH (2014) "Soup consumption is associated with a lower dietary energy density and a better diet quality in US adults." *British Journal of Nutrition 2014 Apr 28: 111(8) 1474-80*

Soup eaters have a lower risk of being overweight

[30] Zhu Y & Hollis JH (2013) "Soup consumption is associated with a reduced risk of overweight and obesity but not metabolic syndrome in US adults" *PLoS One. 2013; 8(9): e75630*

Soup eaters have smaller waists – Fact!

[31] Kuroda M, Ohta M, Okufuji T, Takigami C, Eguchi M, et al. (2011) "Frequency of soup intake is inversely associated with body mass index, waist circumference, and waist-to-hip ratio, but not with other metabolic risk factors in Japanese men. " *Journal of the American Dietetic Association* *111: 137–142*

All types of soup are good for weight loss

[32] Flood JE & Rolls BJ (2007) "Soup preloads in a variety of forms reduce meal energy intake" *Appetite. Nov 2007; 49(3): 626-634*

Don't expect the chia seed to quell your hunger if you eat as you've always eaten

[33] Nieman DC, Cayea EJ, Austin MD, Henson DA, McAnulty SR, Jin F (2009) *"Chia seed does not promote weight loss or alter disease risk factors in overweight adults. "* Nutrition Research. 2009;29:414- 418

That curry can help you to lose weight

[34] Saito M & Yoneshiro T (2013) *"Capsinoids and related food ingredients activating brown fat thermogenesis and reducing body fat in humans"* Current Opinion in Lipidology 2013 Feb 24(1) 71-7

The BMI is pretty poor at diagnosing obesity

[35] Romero-Corral, A; Somers, V K; Sierra-Johnson, J; Thomas, R J; Collazo-Clavell, M L; Korinek, J et al. (2008). "Accuracy of body mass index in diagnosing obesity in the

adult general population". *International Journal of Obesity* **32** (6): 959–66

If you use your willpower it will start to weaken and doesn't work as well the next time you need it

[36] Baumeister, RF (2003) "Ego depletion and self-regulation failure: a resource model of self-control": *Alcoholism Clinical and Experimental Research (2003) Feb 27(2) 281-4*

If you are faced with lots of food - you will lose your self control

[37] Vohs, K.D., & Heatherton, T. F. (2000) "Self-regulatory failure: A resource depletion approach": *Psychological Science, 11* (3), 249–54

You can you train your brain to enjoy healthy foods

[38] Deckersbach T, Das S.K., Urban L.E., Salinardi T, Batra P, Rodman A.M., Arulpragasam A.R., Dougherty D.D, Roberts S.B. (2014) "Pilot randomized trial demonstrating reversal of obesity-related abnormalities in reward system responsivity to food cues with a behavioral intervention". *Nutrition & Diabetes*, 2014; 4 (9): e129